Arab Public Library

20035813

YO-AXE-839

OCT 10 1986
NOV 3 1986
MAR 5 1990

155.646 20035813
KOR Kornheiser, Tony
    The Baby Chase

The Baby Chase

PROPERTY OF
ARAB PUBLIC LIBRARY

The Baby Chase

The Baby Chase
TONY KORNHEISER

Atheneum   New York   1983

Library of Congress Cataloging in Publication Data

Kornheiser, Tony.
　　The baby chase.

　　1. Marriage—United States—Psychological aspects—
Case studies.　2. Childlessness—United States—
Psychological aspects—Case studies.　3. Adoption—
United States—Psychological aspects—Case studies.
4. Black market—United States—Case studies.　I. Title.
HQ536.K67　1983　　　155.6'46　　　82-73025
ISBN 0-689-11354-4

Copyright © 1983 by Anthony I. Kornheiser
All rights reserved
Published simultaneously in Canada by McClelland and Stewart Ltd.
Composed by Westchester Book Composition Inc., Yorktown Heights, New York

Designed by Mary Cregan

*For my father,
and in loving memory of my mother*

Acknowledgments

I want to thank the following people for their special contributions to this book: Harriet Fier, Jane Amsterdam, Shelby Coffey, Carol Weisman, Ben Bradlee, Leslie Scherr, Sterling Lord, and Tom Stewart. And I want especially to thank my wife, Karril, without whose love and support this book could never have been written.

The names and some identifying characteristics of certain people in this book have been changed. The names have been changed to Polly Westin, Grace Zimmer, Judy Amalfitano, W. Allan Cavas, Donna Finnegan, Jeff Lovinger, and Mona Lupica.

The Baby Chase

Wednesday, July 8

Her name was Polly Westin.
She was from Silver Spring, a close-in Maryland suburb.
We didn't know her, but Karril had just been given her name and number by a mutual friend who knew how much we wanted to adopt a child.
Call Polly, Karril was told, she might be able to help.
What the hell, it was a good cause. And a local call.
We finished dinner hurriedly and called. Karril dialed from the phone in the kitchen. I was on the extension in the bedroom, pen in hand, paper in front of me. After eleven years as a newspaper reporter I cannot talk on the phone to anyone, not even my father, without taking notes.
Polly said she'd been expecting our call.
What she said next I am not likely to forget, and not just because I wrote it down, but because it shaped and paced and dominated the course of our lives for the next twelve days. Perhaps it does even now.
Polly said, "I may have a baby for you."

According to government figures, 20 percent of American couples of child-bearing age—six million couples—are infertile.
Infertile *adj.*: not fertile or productive: barren.

3

Wednesday, July 8

Infertility. Lately it's the flavor of the month. You read about it in books. In newspaper and magazine articles. Hear about it on radio call-in shows. See it on made-for-television movies. On public broadcasting specials. On Donahue. It's only a matter of time until it gets the superstar treatment. On Johnny. "You look like a great audience tonight. My producer tells me you're all infertile? Maybe if you went away for a weekend, relaxed. Just a little joke there. I know it's not psychological; I mean if it was all in your head, why would you take off your pants? Do I have this right, there are ten million infertile Americans? Talk about unlucky, how'd you like to have the Pampers route in that neighborhood? All kidding aside, I wish we could get into a serious discussion of your problem, you know, something productive, but we've got a show to do. But look, you've been great sports. I don't want you to leave here empty-handed. Ed, what do we have for all these nice infertile folks? How about some nice Johnny Mathis albums and a home version of 'The Newlywed Game?'"

Infertile. Between inferno and infest.

I want to tell you what it feels like not to be able to have a kid, what it does to your self-esteem and your self-image, not to mention your sex life. What it does to you psychologically, emotionally, even spiritually, to go through nine years of marriage childless. Not productive. Barren. To become progressively more discouraged as you move from fertility specialist to fertility specialist, from basal thermometer chart to blood test to urine test to sperm test to hormone test to mucus test to the ever popular post-coital test, to fertility pills to injections to surgical procedures like the laparoscopy, the open laparoscopy, the hysterosalpingogram, the lysis of adhesions. Day after day, month after month, year

Wednesday, July 8

after year. Nine. Count them. To suffer such profound pain that finally, with no one else to turn to, you turn to each other and wail—why us? Why can't we make a baby? What did we do that was so terrible, so awful, so unspeakably horrible, that God won't let us have a child?

I want to tell you what it feels like to be twenty-five, then twenty-eight, then thirty, then thirty-two, to be trying all this time to have children, because this is all you want from life. Not fame, not fortune, just this one thing—to have a baby—and *still* not have one, and hear the inexorable tick of the biological clock as it grinds you down. To watch in envy as your friends have children. To congratulate them on their good fortune—not meaning a word of it, wishing all the while it was you, not them. Cursing their luck, not just the ones who married six, seven, eight years after you did; at least they wanted kids. No, the ones who said kids were so, you know, *restrictive,* so why have them? And now she's over there by the brie, wine glass in one hand, cigarette in the other, seven months pregnant, looking like she just swallowed Ohio, telling people that "...it was something of an accident, and for sure it will cramp my life style, but look on the bright side, it's a tax deduction and who knows—maybe it will make me settle down." To be able to fake it with everyone but her, so please, *please,* someone have the decency to tell her not to invite us to the baby shower.

I want to tell you what it feels like to listen to the long-distance calls from your aunt that starts out with the weather and how the man who came to hang the new drapes looked just like the Watnicks's idiot boy. And then goes into something like, "...which reminds me, dear, remember little Frannie Besser? When you were home from college she'd come over and you'd help her with biology? Well, she married an oral surgeon, and just last week she had a baby boy. Too soon? What are you talking, too soon? They should all wait as long as you? So when are you going to make your mother happy and give her a grandchild already? Shh, shhhh, I know. Don't you think your mother cries to me? But just this once listen to your old aunt: take a nice trip to the mountains, you and him, go to one of those fancy motels with the bathtubs and the wine and relax."

I want to tell you what it feels like to get the one call you've dreaded above all others, the one from your only sister—your baby sister—and she doesn't quite know how to tell you this, and she's so sorry for your problem, but she and Jack have hopes and dreams of their own, and God, she wishes it was you, but she couldn't keep putting it off, and she understands if you don't feel like singing and dancing about it, but she's pregnant. Okay? Okay? Please say it's okay.

I want to tell you what it feels like to have a visceral reaction to every pregnant woman you see. To go beyond jealousy, to hate, despise, positively loathe them, especially those sixteen-year-old chippies who hang around the Burger King knocked up to beat the band; the ones you hear telling their friends they don't want this kid, they'd do anything to get rid of this kid. But "...put it up for adoption? Give up my own flesh and blood? Are you kidding me?"

I want to tell you what it feels like not to want anything to do with kids, not your friend's kids, not your cousin's kids, not even your own nephew, because they all remind you of your own barrenness. To avoid kids and parents of kids, and places where kids and parents of kids gather, like parks and zoos and playgrounds. Because the feelings of inadequacy and pain are too great, and you're sure you're going to cry, just like you

Wednesday, July 8

started to cry that night in the street when you walked the dog and saw three houses in a row with the garbage neatly arranged to be picked up, and one house had empty cartons of Pampers; one house empty cartons of Luvs; and one house empty cartons of Huggies.

So what happens is you become gradually and increasingly more isolated, even ostracized, because you are the only couple your age without kids. And if you avoid kids and parents of kids, who then are you left with but singles? The circle gets tighter all the time until you feel as if you have been left alone in this category of "Childless Couples," like you're the only two from your high school class who didn't go off to college, and when the old gang gets together none of them has anything in common with you anymore, and the past is just a goodbye.

I want to tell you what it feels like to watch your marriage disintegrate because of the shame and guilt you feel in not being able to conceive. To contemplate divorce so the one of you who can make babies can go out and make some babies, because you have become so warped that you now equate self-worth with pregnancy. To take no joy whatsoever in sex, to never use the phrase "making love" anymore, because what you're doing has nothing to do with love, only performance and function, as if you were being road tested. Maybe this time, if the temperature chart is right, if the cycle is normal, if there is ovulation, if the moon is in the seventh house and Jupiter aligned with Mars, maybe this time you'll get lucky and prove the doctors wrong. Serious business. So just roll on, do it, roll off, and lie still. No harm, no foul.

I want to tell you what it feels like to slow dance on the coals of blind faith and utter despair. To light candles. To pray. To cry yourselves to sleep. To grieve, not

Wednesday, July 8

for the actual child you lost, but for the potential child you'll never have. The broken promise; the shattered dream. To see yourselves growing old and useless, alone together, afraid that some monstrous judgment has been made on you for reasons you cannot even guess, and that the sentence is to be forced to exchange blame and pity for eternity. To think that no matter what else you accomplish in life, it is nothing, and thus, to be ready and willing to do anything to set it right and have a baby. *Anything.*

I want to tell you how it feels to be that desperate.

But I can't; I don't know those words.

I can only tell you that each day you die a little more. You hate yourself a little more. You hate each other a little more until it seems you are consumed with hate, and you are bound by that hate and driven by the relentless treadmill of your failure, and you feed on the conviction that no one can feel your pain, that nothing other than a child can fill the pathetic emptiness of your life.

So when the dream comes, you hold your breath with your eyes closed. And when someone named Polly Westin says she may have a baby for you—but if you are interested there are certain conditions that must be met—you do not ask, what conditions? You say, "Yes. Yes, we are very interested. Thank you, thank you so very much. God bless you."

God bless her.

And God help you. Because if you think the pain is over now, that there are only good times ahead, you are wrong.

God help you, because you are so wrong.

In the next twelve days there would be many, almost daily phone calls to and from Polly Westin, and all, in

Wednesday, July 8

their way, would be riveting. But none so much as this one. The first.

She said she was an adoptive parent herself and that she was part of what sounded like a loose confederation of similar parents "who were simply trying to help other nice young couples adopt children." She said she was "with Gray Market," in a flat, familiar tone, as if it were a common brand name, like Avon or Amway, as if the proper response should be—oh yeah, sure, Gray Market, that's a terrific product you have there. Have you got anything in the eight-pound, five-ounce range with dark hair and blue eyes?

In fact, I had never heard of Gray Market. Nor had Karril.

Polly explained that Gray Market babies were different from Black Market babies. "Black Market babies are totally illegal, because in Black Market you pay a lot of money, maybe $50,000 for a baby. Gray Market is legal because you don't pay nearly as much."

I told her that I thought paying for a baby—no matter how much you paid—was illegal.

She said, "No, believe me, Gray Market is legal. I know it's legal in Maryland. I work for the state, doing adoptions, and we do this all the time. We're people just like you, people who can't have children and wanted them so badly. We've been fortunate enough to adopt, and we want to make it easier for you adopt also. We just help people. But if you don't want to adopt..."

"No." I couldn't say it quickly enough. "No, please. I'm sure it's legal. Please, what do we have to do?"

"I don't have any of the details now. All I can tell you is that I got a call the other day from my contact in New Jersey, a woman with Gray Market up there, and she said she knew of a girl who was about to give birth and couldn't keep the baby. It just wasn't right for

9

Wednesday, July 8

her at this time. She wanted to place the baby out of state. My contact asked if I knew a couple down here who would give the baby a good home, and I immediately thought of you."

Immediately thought of us?

Was this woman for real?

She'd never met us, never even spoken to us before this phone call. How could she know we'd give the baby a good home? How could she know we didn't live in a cave and eat live chickens?

Whatever she knew of us had to have come from Mona Lupica, the mutual friend who'd just called here and told Karril to call Polly. Mona and Polly were in the same cooking club; Mona and Karril were co-workers in a boutique where Karril sold bridal gowns. Assuming that Mona told Polly everything she knew of us, all it could be was that we were in our early thirties, that we had moved to Washington, D.C. from New York, that Karril was quiet and pretty and seemed to like her job, and that I was a writer for the *Washington Post*. You need more information than that to get a library card. I was guessing, but my immediate reaction to Polly's preposterous statement was that whatever the deal was, our entry into it was last-minute.

Karril was downstairs. I couldn't see her, but I knew she was twenty-eight flavors' worth of excited; she hadn't touched her dinner after getting off the phone with Mona, and it was all I could do to get her to let me finish before calling Polly.

Nine years.

Nine years of her refusing to make any friends. Why get involved when she'd only have to drop them as soon as they became pregnant?

Nine years of her drifting from one marginal job to

Wednesday, July 8

another. Why get a career-oriented job when all she wanted as a career was motherhood?

Nine years of her thinking—I am empty without a baby; I am nothing.

I didn't have to be in the room with my wife to know exactly what she was feeling: Oh my God, this is it, this is from heaven. Somebody heard us. This is it.

I knew I shouldn't count on Karril for a lot of objectivity from here on. For nine years she had systematically gone through her life closing all the doors and pulling down the shades. Now, deus ex machina, here is this Polly Westin person throwing open the shutters on a window of opportunity, telling her it's all waiting outside, everything Karril always wanted, tied up in a pink or blue ribbon. Against that what chance did I have of convincing Karril that she ought to put on sunglasses before she looked, in case the light was too strong and it would blind her? Might as well try and catch the wind.

"When is the baby due?" Karril asked.

"It could happen anytime, maybe as soon as tonight," Polly said. "Do you work?"

What an odd question. Didn't she know from Mona?

"Yes. I'm a bridal consultant."

"Of course you'll have to quit your job. You simply must stay home and raise the child. We won't give you the baby unless you stay home with it."

"I want to stay home and raise the child. I want to be a full-time mother. Do you want me to quit tomorrow?"

"No, you can wait until you get the baby. But then you must quit your job."

Then Polly paused: "Now," she said, "what I need to know is, how fast can you get the money?"

I had been waiting for the money to come up. The

Wednesday, July 8

baby was the carrot, the money was the stick.

"How much money?" I asked.

"I don't know for sure, but would it be a problem for you to come up with $15,000?"

I didn't hesitate. "No problem at all."

The number was discouraging, but not surprising. We'd never heard the $50,000 figure Polly quoted for a Black Market baby; we'd heard that healthy white infants brought as much as $30,000. But while $15,000 seemed cheap in comparison, it was hard to imagine that such a fee was within legal limits. Trying to give Polly every benefit of the doubt, I wondered if she'd simply thrown out that number to see how we'd react. If that kind of money was no problem, she might conclude we were in a financial position to ensure that the baby had a good home. I hoped she was trying to gauge us, not gouge us.

"How soon can you get it?"

I wanted her to think money was no object. "How soon do you want it?"

"Can you have it on hand by tomorrow?"

"Cash or check?"

"Cash—it's for your own protection."

"We can have it tomorrow."

"Good. That's what I needed to know. I'll call my contact in New Jersey and tell her I've found a couple, and recommend she accept you. In the meantime, don't tell anyone about this. No one." Her business done, Polly abruptly changed her tone. Had she been a car, she'd have dropped her transmission from the sudden shift. "Well, it was wonderful meeting you. Congratulations. I just know this is all going to work out. And let me tell you as an adoptive mother myself, once you hold that baby in your arms it'll be yours as much as if you had given birth to it yourself."

Wednesday, July 8

Her words were coated with stardust. *Once you hold that baby in your arms it'll be yours as much as if you had given birth to it yourself.*

Karril took the steps two at a time.
"Well, what do you think?" she asked.
"No, no. First you," I said.
Karril had never been verbal enough to please either of us. We'd met at a summer camp where we both worked as counselors, and on one of our first dates she compared us to Henry Higgins and Eliza Doolittle. She said most people thought she was shy, but the real reason she was so quiet was because she never had anything to say, so could I please teach her to be more of a conversationalist? I'd been attracted to her looks; she'd obviously been attracted to my mouth. But okay. Sure. If she wanted me to water and nurture and cultivate her until she blossomed into a Dorothy Parker, fine; if she believed in that kind of magic, fine; if she thought that just by standing near my shoes she'd eventually grow my feet, fine.

For a long time I ignored the fact that it wasn't working because I not only had a beautiful girl hanging on my arm, but on my every word as well. And I grew to love her in spite of—maybe even because of—her quietness. There was such a softness to her, such a tenderness. I felt calmer just being around her; I felt better for her nearness. She rounded off my edges. And if the truth be told, there was also a helplessness in her manner that appealed to me. I could be her rock and her redeemer. But as years passed the conversation gap widened, and although we could have easily bridged the distance with words, she stopped using them. I sometimes thought that Karril turned inward like that to punish both of us for crimes of greater and lesser articulation—that she used

Wednesday, July 8

her silence as a weapon. In any case, the spoken word became a fault line that often rumbled beneath us. And so, before I said anything that could influence Karril's stance, I wanted her to tell me exactly how she felt about this situation. Not so much for my benefit, as hers. I didn't want to drown her out. I just wanted her to hear herself say it. So there would be no mistakes later. So it would be on the record.

"I'm stunned."

"Stunned?"

"Yeah, stunned. Euphoric. What do you want from me? You know all the words."

"Sorry. Go ahead."

"This is what I've been waiting for all these years. And it's happening now, it's actually happening. Everything is over with now—that wanting and not having, those feelings of inadequacy, not being like the rest of the girls because I don't have a baby carriage. All those feelings are just out the window."

Her face was a book, open to the page where the sun finally breaks through the thick, dark clouds and shines directly, and only, on the young lovers. She was beaming, on the verge of crying from joy. The sight of Karril like this took my breath away; I wished I could wrap myself around her now and keep it like this forever. I could remember seeing her like this only once, that day five years ago when she found out that she was finally pregnant, when this laboratory test, unlike all the many others, was positive. That was the happiest day of our lives. Short and sweet. The following day Karril started staining, and her doctor told her she'd suffered a spontaneous abortion. She had never conceived again.

I kicked myself for what I was about to do, and I did it anyway.

I made myself into stone.

Wednesday, July 8

"I don't think it would be wise to get carried away." I looked directly into her eyes and watched them deflate, like soufflés, from the thrust of the words. "I know it's easy for me to say that. I know you think I'm hiding behind my work personality, and refusing to get emotionally involved, and maybe I am. But one of us has to. Grant me that. And look, I've obviously been trained to look at these things more objectively than you."

"These *things?*" She came at me like an avalanche. "What things? I'm talking about a baby. We've waited nine years for a baby, and now we can get one. So don't give me this 'these things' crap. How do you feel about this baby?"

The unexpected violence of her reaction knocked me back on my heels. I took a moment to gather myself: "I'll tell you. But don't you yell at me, okay? Because all that does, your yelling, is prove my point that you can't be rational about this. So don't yell." Then I came out counterpunching: "Now how do I feel about this baby? First of all, I feel it's illegal. I don't know what the hell Gray Market is, but if the difference between it and Black Market is just the amount of money being passed under the table, then it's clear to me it's a scam. It's selling a baby. Second of all, who the hell is this woman? How do we know if she's legit? Who is she kidding, telling us she 'immediately thought' of us? She never even met us. You want to open yourself up to more hurt? I mean, haven't we been hurt enough not being able to have kids? Third of all, what's this New Jersey contact hocus-pocus?"

I stopped for breath, but I wasn't through yet. Not by a long shot. Even if Karril had wanted to get a word in edgewise, she wouldn't have had a prayer. I was on a roll: "Karril, we don't know a damned thing about what's going on here, except what some total stranger

Wednesday, July 8

tells us. We're being rushed, and we're being manipulated. All she gave a damn about was whether we could come up with the money. And even if that's just a ballpark figure, it's a pretty fancy ballpark. Do you have any idea how long it took me to save $15,000? Do you know how much we'd have left if we spent it? About a buck three-eighty is how much. And cash yet. All cash. *'For your protection.'* Give me a break. How are we protected? They want cash so they can take the money and run, and we won't be able to prove a damned thing. And why'd she tell us not to tell anyone? If it was so legitimate, why'd she make it seem like the whole deal ought to take place underneath the 59th Street Bridge at four in the morning?"

I was pacing the floor, wearing a groove in the carpet. My frenzy had chased the dog from the room and all but nailed Karril to her chair. I tried to calm down, but it was impossible. There was still thunder in the air, still rain in the clouds: "I swear, Karril, this thing has shuck written all over it. God only knows where the money's going. How much to Polly? How much to this New Jersey contact, who, may I add, still has to approve us? How much to the girl? I assume they have a lawyer. How much to him? How many people ultimately get rich off our suffering? Look, I want a kid every bit as much as you do, but I don't want to get kicked in the stomach for my trust. I'm not saying I won't go through with this, but I'm saying that before we do anything, before we sign anything, and especially before we *hand over* anything, we ought to think about this whole deal, think it over more carefully than we've ever thought anything over before. I collect facts, Kar; I'm useless without facts. So look, I want you to take notes every time you speak to this Polly Westin woman. Real, live, written notes. And if she has you speak to anyone else

Wednesday, July 8

involved in this, you take notes on those conversations too. I'll make a leg man out of you yet. In the meantime I'll start calling lawyers to see what Gray Market is all about, and whether it's kosher. But the crucial thing is not to be rushed. And to start assembling the facts. Okay?"

"So you don't trust her?"

"I can't get anything past you, can I? In a word, no."

"And that's why you took notes?"

"Yeah."

"Can I see them?"

"Here."

I gave them to her, and her eyes immediately focused on the bottom of the envelope I was using as a legal pad. Right to where I had been jotting baby names.

"Baby names? I thought you were taking notes, Mr. Ace Reporter. Mr. Objectivity. I thought you didn't want to get emotionally involved?"

She was laughing.

"So I lied. So sue me."

"You really do want a baby, don't you?"

"More than I want you to know. Maybe more than I want me to know."

"So we go ahead with it?"

"Of course we do. What choice do we have?"

In 1975, a survey by the East-West Population Institute revealed the five most common answers given by parents to the question "Why did you have children?" The answers, in order, were: "I don't know"; "A general liking for children"; "It's instinctive, natural to have children"; "To continue the family name"; "To please other people, like grandparents."

It bears repeating: the most common answer was "I don't know."

17

Wednesday, July 8

We knew.

I almost hesitate to explain why we wanted a child, because it seems it should be so evident, and to analyze it, to put it under a microscope and examine it, risks distorting it; you put a butterfly wing under a microscope and its fine, thin veins appear like troughs.

Yes, we wanted a child because we had a general liking for children. Yes, we wanted a child because it seemed instinctive to have one. Yes, we wanted a child to continue the family name. Yes, we wanted a child to please others as well as ourselves. It's perfectly normal to want a child because of how it will make you feel. If a by-product of having a child is that you feel better about yourselves, more comfortable, more connected with the world around you, good. Why not?

We wanted a child for the same reasons, right or wrong, as fertile couples want children—because it seemed good, because it seemed right, because it seemed natural. We wanted to raise someone. To give a child a home and a value system, and watch it grow up and take its place in the world. We wanted to be part of something larger than ourselves. Our grandparents had our parents, our parents had us. It's all of a piece. That's why they call it the biological chain. We wanted to add a link.

We were two, and we wanted to be three.

We were a couple, and we wanted to be a family.

We were full, and there was much we had to give. Yet we were empty, and there was much we had to gain.

We wanted a child for the best reason on earth. To love.

It was important to me that my father be the first to know, and I immediately called him in Fort Lauderdale. My mother had died of cancer a few years earlier, just

Wednesday, July 8

three months after they moved from Long Island to Florida to retire; now there was just my Dad and me. He had been a prince about grandchildren, or his lack thereof. Recognizing what a sensitive area it was for Karril and me, he never brought up the subject of our infertility. But he was past seventy now, and although he wouldn't say so for fear of hurting my feelings, he wanted very much to be a grandfather. For all the standard, time-honored reasons. Everyone his age seemed to be a grandparent, and he wanted to be one too; he wanted the pleasure of doting on a grandchild, of buying presents and showing off baby pictures; he wanted to be able to join in on the major topic of conversation at his retirement condominium; he wanted to see his line continue. Can you blame him? And even more than he wanted it for himself, he wanted it for his only child.

I told him all about the conversation with Polly Westin, how strange a setup it seemed and how nervous it made me. Then I told him that Karril and I were going along with it, at least temporarily, until we had enough facts to make a reasonable decision.

"So I'm calling because I want to know how you feel about us adopting."

Which wasn't quite true. I already knew. I wanted to give him the chance to say it. A study by the sociologist David Kirk showed that 20 percent of prospective grandparents at first reacted negatively to adoption plans. My father was in this group. Whenever I brought it up he would tell me the story of the people he knew who had adopted years ago. And once again he repeated it now:

"For a while everything was fine with the boy, but you can't control genetics," my father said. "By the time the boy was seven or eight, what he really was began to show. His natural parents were very poor, real peasant stock; the boy obviously inherited their characteristics."

Wednesday, July 8

I'd heard the story enough to know there was no shaking my father from this tree. So rather than futilely object on the grounds of extreme prejudice, I let him continue: "By the time he was ten he was getting into all sorts of trouble in the neighborhood; he was shoplifting and bullying younger kids and he was doing badly in school. You can imagine what a heartache it was becoming for his parents. They did everything they could. They took him to counselors. They got him tutors. Really, they gave him a much better home than he deserved. But he didn't appreciate it. When he was sixteen he just ran away. They never saw him again. I would have said, good riddance. Who needs a child like that? But the mother still cries. I wouldn't want you to make a mistake like that. If you and Karril can't have children, so be it. But this adoption? Well, I just don't think you can be too sure."

He meant well, and I loved him. But I had to try and persuade him that his example was the exception, not the rule.

"Dad, you're telling me it's a crapshoot. I know it's a crapshoot. But it's a crapshoot even with your own. Look at me, I'm six feet tall. You're five-six, Mom was five-four. Where'd I get the height? From the milkman? No. From some recessive trait. Now what if you were carrying some recessive trait for mental retardation? Or a fatal disease?"

"But I wasn't."

"Not with me, maybe. But you didn't have any other children. Forget about you. How do we know I'm not carrying some genetic time bomb that I'd pass along? How can you prevent something crazy from happening during a pregnancy? Let's say Mom had eaten some kind of weird fish when she was pregnant, and the mercury level in it made me deformed? I reminded him that the

Wednesday, July 8

year before, my cousin Shelley had given birth to a child with a severely cleft palate. Nothing like that had ever happened in her family or her husband's. Their first child, Nathan, had been born perfectly healthy. "I was down there visiting you the day Seth was born, remember?"

"I took you to the hospital."

"Right. We went to the hospital, and saw him in the nursery. He had no lips. There was just that big hole from the bottom of his nose to his chin."

"You should see him now. The surgeons did a remarkable job. If you didn't know, you couldn't tell."

"Thank God for reconstructive plastic surgery. But my point is, Dad, that it can happen to anyone. Are there better, more devoted parents in the world than Shelley and Arthur? No, but it happened to them, and nobody yet knows why. So it doesn't just happen when you adopt. I think how you raise a kid counts for more than what's in there before you get him. Look, if it'll make you feel better, if they offer us a peasant baby I won't take it unless they promise me he'll be able to root out truffles with his nose."

"Have it your way. Be a wise guy."

"Dad, I'm just trying to say that not every adoption has to be the horror story that one was."

"You asked me how I felt. I told you. I just want to save you some pain."

"I appreciate that, but there's more pain in not having any kids. This may be our last shot."

"You don't know that."

"No, I don't. But it's been nine years. For as long as I've been married you've been telling me that it took you and Mom eight years to have me, and that she almost died during delivery. Dad, we caught you and passed you. Shouldn't we read the writing on the wall?"

21

Wednesday, July 8

"You know I'm sorry for you."

"I know, and I appreciate that you never bring it up. But we have this opportunity now, and I want to know something. Will you love this child if we get it? Will you be its grandfather?"

"Of course I will." There were tears gathering in his voice. "I'd be proud to be its grandfather. And no matter what you do, I'm proud of you, son. I love you."

"I love you too." There was one more thing. I took a deep breath. "I was thinking of naming the baby after Mom." God, this was harder than I thought. "I won't do it without your permission."

"I never told you how much your mother wanted to be a grandmother. It was her only regret." His tears were almost choking him; I was crying just listening to him. "She had a full life, Tony. We did it all. We traveled all around the world. Europe, South America, Asia. And we always went first class, you know that. We were married thirty-seven years. We had you, and you turned out so well. But she wanted to be a grandmother. I'd be very proud if you named the baby after her, and I'm sure wherever she is now, she's very proud that you would do that."

Evan, if it was a boy.

Elizabeth, if it was a girl.

Karril and I had already decided on those names.

"You know," my father said, suddenly very cheerful, "this baby could be born on your birthday."

My birthday, July 13, was just five days away.

"Wouldn't that be something," I said. What I didn't tell him was that I prayed that wouldn't happen. If it did, then come hell or high water I'd be locked into this adoption. Because that would be a divine sign.

When I got off the phone with my father I had Karril call her parents, who also lived in Fort Lauderdale, hav-

Wednesday, July 8

ing moved there from New York about a year and a half earlier. They could easily afford to be selective about adoption; their other child, Pamela, three years younger than Karril, had given birth to a son in February. But even if they'd had no grandchildren I'd have expected a lukewarm reaction. I vaguely remembered a conversation we'd had in which Karril's parents took the position that having a baby was God's will, and that, God willing, we'd have one someday. But I could be wrong on that because over the years our conversations tended to be few and far between; we'd all agreed that we got along best when we talked least.

As it turned out, Karril's mother wasn't against adoption. In fact, had it not been for the delicacy of the subject, she might have suggested it to Karril long ago. But Karril's mother was hesitant about *this* adoption. She didn't mention genes, but she worried about the timing and the money. Everything seemed so rushed. If it was happening so fast, she reasoned, it couldn't be good. And it seemed like so much money. Better to adopt through an agency than a phone call, she said.

We didn't start off thinking adoption. Adoption was for those unfortunate people who couldn't have their own children; we intended to. But after years of failing we reluctantly concluded it might be impossible for us, and began thinking about alternative ways to become parents.

We had heard about catching lightning in a bottle. About how some couples get lucky when priests or obstetricians, or others with access to and influence with a pregnant girl, get her to agree to place her baby with a couple they know. If that happened, great, we'd take it. But it was a real long shot. We weren't Catholic, so

Wednesday, July 8

the priest was out. But we were Jewish, so we knew a lot of doctors.

We discounted the sci-fi methods of creating a child, both the *in vitro* or "test-tube" fetilization, and the independent contracting of a "surrogate mother" to carry the child produced by her egg being artificially inseminated with my sperm. At the time we were considering alternatives the only *in vitro* work was being done in England. And where were we going to get a surrogate? Were we supposed to take out an ad in *Hustler*?

We decided that the most accessible and logical route was to adopt someone else's child and raise it as our own. One less child goes unloved; one less infertile couple goes unfulfilled. A good trade for both teams. What kind of child was never an issue. We wanted a white infant. Perhaps if we already had a couple of kids we would have been receptive to adopting an older child or "special needs" child, the umbrella designation for children with all manner of handicaps. We weren't so noble. When the time came, we would want to replicate the biological process of parenting as closely as possible.

We plead guilty to wanting the child we couldn't have.

We didn't know the mechanics of getting one, but we didn't think it would be too difficult. From all we gathered in the media, teenage pregnancies were about as common as brown sauce on egg foo young. Assuming the adoption agencies were looking for couples like us— educated, affluent, settled—we anticipated phoning for an appointment, going down to the agency to sign up, sitting through an amicable interview, then waiting a couple of months until the call came that we ought to spruce up the crib because our child was waiting. Seriously, how tough could it be?

Very tough.

We had no idea that the demand was so large. Or

Wednesday, July 8

that the supply was so small, so very small. Smaller, as it were, than a baby's tiny toes. A seller's market.

Because there are no federal statutes regulating adoption, all record keeping is done by the individual states as each sees fit. And because the prevailing social priority is to ensure privacy, what records that are kept tend to be superficial. For example, more than half of all adoptions are known to be between relatives, typically the legal adoption of stepchildren. But there are no reliable statistical breakdowns of the age, sex, race, or religion of adopted children.

Yet even with this caveat that collective national statistics are not based on uniform data, it is instructive that Senator Jeremiah Denton, chairman of the Senate subcommittee on Aging, Family, and Human Services, reported: total adoptions may have declined by as much as 50 percent in the decade of the 1970s. The largest intramural decline occurred in the area of adoptions of nonrelatives, typically the adoption of illegitimate, unwanted children. In 1979 only 22,000 infants were available for adoption.

Six million infertile couples.

Twenty-two thousand adoptable infants.

Where have all the babies gone?

Contraception. It's a chicken-and-egg call on which came first, the sexual revolution or the pill. But by the 1970s sophisticated methods of contraception were readily available, and teenagers were being encouraged to avail themselves of them, in many cases by parents, teachers, and clergy. The bedrock rationale behind contraception has always been planned parenthood.

Abortion. In 1973 the United States Supreme Court ruled that no state may deny a woman's rights to abortion at the initial stages of pregnancy. This is after-the-fact contraception. The National Committee for Adoption reported that in 1978 approximately 434,000 teenaged girls elected to have abortions. Teenaged girls statistically prefer abortion to carrying to term by a ratio of three to one.

Parenting. This is the big one. Even with sophisticated contraception and abortion on demand, almost 600,000 children—17 percent of total births—are born out of wedlock each year. Teenagers account for 45 percent of those illegitimate births, and in 1978 fully 96 percent of those teenagers chose to keep their babies.

Attitude. Recent social and cultural experience conspires against encouraging unwed mothers to choose the adoption option. The prevalent belief in the indomitability of flesh and blood has fostered the notion that the natural mother is the best person to raise her child, no matter how ill-equipped she may be emotionally or financially. Senator Denton reported "strong peer pressure is erroneously instilling the belief that giving your baby up for adoption is a cruel punishment for the baby." The prejudice of the courts, the counselors and, increasingly, the clergy is toward keeping the biological chain intact, and is, therefore, necessarily anti-adoption. The Women's Movement has been a serious force in influencing women to think more confidently about their abilities to raise their children alone. The rise in the divorce rate and the increase in single-parent households—20 percent of white children and 50 percent of black children now live in single-parent households—help reduce the stigma of raising illegitimate children, as does the rise in government welfare "entitlement" programs. Obviously, the Victorian concept of sin has been inverted. It used to be that the sin was having the baby out of wedlock. Now the sin is giving that baby away. And what you get is children raising children.

So, facing a bottom line of 6,000,000 infertile couples

Wednesday, July 8

and 22,000 adoptable babies, where can you go?

You can go to your state's public adoption agencies that consider you a constituent. You may be eligible for service from city, county, and state agencies. If you are flexible, willing to adopt an older and/or special-needs child, you can almost walk out the door a parent; public agencies are top-heavy with children nobody seems to want. If you are inflexible, insistent on a healthy white infant, bring a lot of change for the meter, because even after you're placed at the end of the waiting list the routine waiting time at a public adoption agency for such a child is at least five years—if they get any white infants, which they often do not. The District of Columbia's Department of Social Services, for example, said it hadn't had a single white infant to place in four years. Waiting list gridlock. Sorry.

You can go to a private adoption agency. They regularly get more white infants, so their waiting time can be substantially less, maybe as little as eighteen months to two years—if the agency agrees to work with you. William Pierce, president of the National Committee for Adoption, an organization funded by many of the largest private adoption agencies in the country, generally advises prospective adopters that "if you are pleasantly and aggressively persistent you will be successful in finding an appropriate agency to work with you within five years."

In the meantime, unlike a public agency, a private agency can reject an applicant with impunity: Most commonly the waiting list is closed; no new names are being added this year, or next year, or in the foreseeable future. Or the interview doesn't go well; you are perceived as too aggressive, too passive, too rigid, too bending. Or you're the wrong religion; or you're not rich enough; or you're not moral enough. Or you fail their home study.

Wednesday, July 8

No agency, public or private, hands over a child without the adoptive parents first passing a "home study," an investigation into parental fitness by a licensed social worker. It's a painful irony that the only people who have to pass a test certifying them for parenting are the infertile.

Or you can go overseas. An increasing number of adoptive parents get children from foreign countries, notably Colombia and Mexico. In the 1970s United States citizens adopted 30,000 foreign-born children; in 1981 alone there were 8,000 such adoptions. There are agencies in the United States that specialize in international adoptions. The children are available, and it can be done quickly. But when horror stories about international adoption are told they are invariably about the health of the children; either an unhealthy child is handed over, or the child's medical history is incomplete and/or fraudulent.

Or you can go through a third party, most frequently a lawyer, but often a doctor or clergyman, who facilitates what is called a private or independent adoption—if such an arrangement is legal in your jurisdiction. In some states, such as Connecticut, Delaware, Massachusetts, Michigan, Minnesota, and North Dakota, it is not. Cynthia D. Martin, in her book *Beating the Adoption Game*, writes that "Adoption agencies over the years have attempted to have private adoptions ruled illegal...they cut into their business." While the agency lobby has been a factor, the fundamental social principle behind the laws forbidding independent adoption is that the potential for abuse is clearly present because the independent process does not provide sufficient protection for the child; prospective adopters aren't subject to the same kind of screening procedures as in agency adoptions. Often the only qualification for getting a child through

Wednesday, July 8

a third party is the ability to meet the financial arrangements. But independent adoption is the route of choice for couples who have been rejected or frustrated by the agencies or the interminable wait for a healthy white infant. And, according to Jacqueline Hornor Plumez in her book *Successful Adoption,* birth mothers choose these adoptions for a variety of reasons: "Many need to have their medical and/or living expenses paid during pregnancy. Most agencies do not provide full payment for medical expenses and often can only suggest welfare as a means of support. Some birth mothers want to...work with a go-between who will allow them to select between the biographies of several [adopters]. Finally, some birth mothers want to avoid agencies because they do not want to participate in the intense counselling agencies give." Parenthetically, some especially want to avoid Catholic and Fundamentalist affiliated agencies so they don't face daily confrontation with the pervasive concept of original sin. While independent adoption may seem like just the ticket, the obstacles are in finding a third party with access to birth mothers, then making certain all parties act legally and responsibly.

Or, if it happens to you like it happened to us—and you have no prior knowledge of any of this—you can go to the telephone and call Polly Westin.

We got into bed. We didn't speak. We didn't touch. For hours we just lay still, questions rolling and tumbling like dice in our heads.

Was this legitimate?
Was it some sort of Byzantine sick joke?
Was it possible to simply dial-a-baby?
Was it a divine test of our righteousness?
Was it Granada, or just Asbury Park?
For the next twelve days Karril and I were under siege.

Wednesday, July 8

Until the deed was done she slept poorly, if at all. She became increasingly silent and withdrawn, turning her anger inward until it bored yet another hole in a colon that after ten years of colitis already resembled a slice of Swiss cheese. I had no problem sleeping; my problem was the recurrent chest pain I had when awake. Anxieties overwhelmed me and made me manic. I threw myself into work, then threw myself at my wife when I got home. While I was intolerant and confrontational, Karril was passive and distant. Our marriage nearly collapsed under the strain, each of us, separately, coming within a moment, a phrase, a shadow of walking. We lied to ourselves, and we lied to each other.

I confess that from the moment I got on the telephone with Polly Westin I imagined myself part of a Greek tragedy. Instead of thrilling me with anticipation, her offer terrified me. I saw whatever control I had over my own life slipping away from me, laughing as it fell. Even in the July swamp-dog heat of Washington, D.C., I felt a chill in my bones, and as I looked for the light at the end of the tunnel, I shivered to think it was attached to an oncoming train that had my name on it.

Thursday, July 9

I liked morning. I liked getting into the day while it was still clean. Over the years, admittedly, I'd become obsessive about my morning routine, but it pleased me to awaken by seven, walk the dog, work up a sweat doing my exercises, take a shower, and then squeeze myself a glass of fresh grapefruit juice.

Responsibility. Sacrifice. Vitamin C.

I mean, how suburbanly virtuous can you get?

Karril seemed allergic to morning. On days when she didn't have to get up for work, she'd sleep so late that I was only half kidding when my first words to her were, "Hi, ready for dinner?" Workdays she'd get on her feet, but between eight and eleven she wasn't just groggy, she was zombified; the only people less alert were plugged into life-support systems.

So, borrowing a philosophy from the back of a cornflakes box, I'd say, "Karril, you can't get up at eight half the time and two the other half. If I showed you a graph of your sleeping patterns it'd look like an outline of the Rocky Mountains. Your life's too chaotic this way. Look, give me two weeks in which you get up every day at seven with me. We'll do some stretching exercises together; you'll get some muscle tone. Then you'll eat a good, hearty breakfast. Two weeks, and I promise you'll

Thursday, July 9

feel better than you ever have in your life, and you'll develop a positive mental attitude."

She would suffer me by listening, affirm the theory, and even agree to try it. Then, two days later, she'd be sleeping until two again. It took me years to understand that Karril hated getting up because she felt she had nothing to get up for as long as she was childless. She slept to escape the emptiness of her life.

At first I was inclined to let her sleep, to allow her that small comfort, even if it seemed an overload of self-pity to lie in bed and put your life on hold so deliberately. Later though, I came to see Karril's protracted sleep as a subconscious indictment of our infertile marriage, and it pained me to see her lying in bed.

I bring this up because Thursday night Karril worked late and therefore wasn't due in until twelve-thirty. Typically, this meant that communication between us was unthinkable until noon, since she'd have the covers over her head. But because I wanted to make sure she understood precisely how I wanted us to proceed with our adoption strategy, I woke her and set out the day's agenda, much like a high school teacher announcing the homework. I went so far as to suggest that Karril take written notes on what I was saying. If looks could kill, I'd be a long time dead.

We would tell no one who didn't need to know. Since both parents already knew, the only other family member who should know this early was Karril's sister, Pamela. Karril would tell no one at work. It was too risky. The day before we picked up the baby she would quit her job, giving no notice. I had no doubt that if she told them earlier she'd be fired. Because my job paid so much more, and the Washington Post Company was infinitely more humane in its labor-management relations, I would tell my immediate editors today, so I could arrange for

Thursday, July 9

the leave time I would need. Others, such as lawyers, advisers, and friends whose support we would need, would be told as the situation required. I assumed that the suspicious nature of the adoption, and her complicity in it, were why Polly told us not to tell anyone; we weren't so much following her dictum as heeding our own fears.

I got to work by nine-thirty. I had a story to write about a national accordion competition and convention in Washington. I'd done the bulk of the reporting the day before, and fortunately the hotel where the competition was ongoing was just around the corner from the *Post*; I could write my scene piece on the ins and outs of these accordionists and still be able to zip over and punch in a few last-minute lines on the eventual champions.

Before I sat down to type though, I told people who would need to know now about the possibility of the adoption—Shelby Coffey, then overall editor of "Style," the section where I wrote, and Jane Amsterdam, my assignment editor. They were good friends, and they unhesitatingly pledged all their help and support; whatever I needed, I had. It didn't surprise me that each was skeptical about the adoption as I outlined it; sometimes I think equal portions of fluoride and skepticism are pumped into the water supply at a newspaper. But I did find it interesting that each offered essentially the same advice: "Be very careful. You ought to allow that behind that façade is a sensitive person, and that you can be psychologically scarred by a disappointment here. And surely Karril, if she wants this child as desperately as you say, is even more vulnerable than you. Make sure you're not doing this in desperation, and make sure you leave yourselves room to maneuver. Tony, you're a high-strung guy to begin with. By the end of this, if you're not careful, you could be a basket case. Maybe for your own good, for some peace of mind, you ought to work real hard every day. Don't work on anything long, no projects. Just do the day hits. Keep them short and funny. Face a deadline three or four times a week and you won't have all that down time when all you'll do is sit and think and drive yourself crazy. Hard work will serve you best."

I knew they were right. I should try and keep busy. And then, when I wasn't writing or reporting, I could use the phones on whatever calls were necessary to the adoption. I made a note to myself to make sure to lower my voice whenever I made an adoption call. Because I thought I was funnier than exploding golf balls, I normally made my phone conversations into auditions for the main room at the Tropicana; I'd have to guard against that now. If anybody noticed my unusual reserve, I'd tell them I was working on a mime act.

I knew we'd eventually need a lawyer in D.C. to handle the adoption, but first I needed general counsel to find out if this thing could possibly be legal. My cousin Shelley's husband, Arthur, was a lawyer in Florida, and I called him at his office. Although they were younger than us, Karril and I felt closer to Shelley and Arthur than to any of our other cousins. They were smart and sweet and loving and, above all, terrific parents. Knowing how disappointed we were at not having children, they'd tactfully mentioned adoption, how we ought to consider it. Because it seemed so much easier to do in Florida than in Washington, they'd encouraged us to adopt there, and offered to help us with the process.

I told Arthur I would do nothing to jeopardize his standing within the bar; I simply wanted to know all

Thursday, July 9

the options and inherent risks in this kind of adoption. He didn't know the specific statutes that applied in Washington, but it seemed to him that the money Polly mentioned was high enough to indicate the possible illegality of this transaction. He did not think there could be payment beyond reasonable medical fees for the natural mother's hospitalization—no full support during her pregnancy—and reasonable legal fees for whoever did the paperwork. Since we weren't working through an adoption agency, we couldn't even justify a bureaucratic fee.

"So that's why they want cash, right?" I asked.

"Right," he said. "With cash they can hide any payment above the allowable standard. The other thing you have to worry about from the sound of this is the appearance of coercion. Not only would a large payment make it seem like the mother was coerced into giving up the child, which is illegal, but you have to make sure that the mother can't come back and claim she was coerced into giving up the child for any other reason."

"Like what?"

"Let's say a natural mother wants to reopen an adoption. She goes to court and tells the judge the only reason she gave up her baby in the first place was because her priest told her it was the right thing to do. Now she wants the baby back. The judge might be persuaded to reopen the case on the grounds of coercion; the adoption can be voidable. Even two or three years later they could remove the baby from the adoptive parents. It has happened, and it's devastating."

I felt myself shudder.

The Baby Lenore Case. 1971. New York City. It was all over the papers for weeks. Nick DeMartino, a lawyer, and his wife, Jean, had already adopted once from the prestigious Spence-Chapin child welfare agency in Manhattan. Lenore was their second child from there. The girl's natural mother, a Colombian national named Olga Scarpetta, had signed the surrender decree, legally relinquishing custody of the child to the agency, which had, in turn, given her to the DeMartinos. Months went by, and then Olga Scarpetta sued the agency and went to court claiming she had changed her mind and had been coerced into giving up her baby. Ultimately, the United States Supreme Court refused to overturn a New York State Court of Appeals decision directing the DeMartinos to give baby Lenore back to Olga Scarpetta. But by then the DeMartinos were long gone. They had fled to Florida where a lower court found in their favor. They're still there. Baby Lenore is in the history books. Soon she'll be a teenager.

"There's no protection?" I asked Arthur.

"Not in an illegal adoption. But by the same token, these adoptions happen all the time, and they go through cleanly. Couples know the risks involved, and they choose to take them. And believe me, once they put that baby in your arms it's like he's your natural child, and you'll kill to keep him."

The Baby Lenore memory had gotten to me. I tried to calm myself by talking, but I'm sure it sounded like babble. "We'll tell him he's adopted. We'll tell him before he goes to school so he'll understand."

"I'm sure you'll handle it right."

"Oh, and we'll help him even if he wants to find his biological parents, even at the risk of the enormous hurt that kind of search could cause us. We've talked about it. We'll do it." What the hell was I talking about? Briefly, it occurred to me that I was like a fighter who'd taken a hard right flush on the chin, and was backpedalling around the ring, just trying to stay out of reach until he

Thursday, July 9

could clear his head. I heard Arthur more distinctly now.

"Don't worry about that now. You've got years to worry about that."

"Right." Still shaking away the shadows.

"Anyway, very few adopted children even care to know. It's enough for them that you've chosen them and loved them and made them your own."

I was calm now.

"Arthur, what would you do? Would you take the risk?"

"I don't know what I'd do if I were you. We've been very fortunate in having two children. I can tell you that I have no problems with the morality of this adoption. I think you'd make wonderful parents and I know how hard it is to adopt conventionally. I know how long the lines are, and how difficult an agency can make it on you. I had to tell you the absolute worst that could happen in a situation like this. But I want to do some research into it. Maybe there's a way to do it this way and still have it totally legal. There very well could be. And I think in any case a judge might think twice before taking a baby out of a good home regardless of the legal provocation. If you want the child badly enough, you might want to go ahead with it. Just make sure to get as much information about the child as possible. That's crucial, knowing all you can about medical history. And don't get too nervous. The laws where you live may well be different."

"Thanks, Arthur." Now for the hard part. "Look, I'm not trying to make this into a Robert Ludlum novel, but just for a while can we keep this whole thing between us? Could I possibly invoke attorney-client privilege and ask you not to tell Shelley about this yet? Okay?"

I thought sure I heard him sigh.

"If that's what you want." He was so suddenly flattened. I winced thinking of him as a tire punctured by the force of my request.

"Just for a while. Thanks."

Now I had an educated guess by an educated man that cast at least reasonable doubt as to the legality of Polly Westin's proposal because of the large sum of money involved. That meant that when we went to court to finalize the adoption, if we failed to disclose the full amount we paid in order to ensure the validity of the adoption, we might be committing perjury. And even if we were successful in keeping the sum hidden, and the judge granted the decree, what was to stop the biological mother one, two, five, ten years down the road from seeking a reversal? What if she knocked on the judge's chambers, asking the musical question—"What's an eight-letter word meaning, 'I Want My Kid Back?' You got it, Your Honor. Now sing along with Mama: 'That old coercion up and down my spine/That old coercion when your cash met mine.'"

So those were the risks.

Lots of people take them; we could too.

After all those years of seeing only the side I chose to show the rest of the world, of watching me, Mr. Big Deal Reporter, walk that walk and talk that talk, Arthur probably figured me for a pair of balls the size of Bermuda onions; some pissant thing like an illegal adoption wouldn't even raise a welt. When the time came, I'd just announce, "If not me, who? If not now, when?" Then I'd strap them on and go out into the street and scare the horses.

I wondered if he had any idea how frightened I was. If he had any clue how hollow it was inside the shell. The truth was, when the wind blew, if you listened carefully, you could hear my bluffs rattle. I wasn't a risk

Thursday, July 9

taker. Risks were an extension of the unknown. I was a fact gatherer; I lived in fear of the unknown. Look at the kind of things I'm afraid of: Afraid to fly, afraid of the dark, afraid of water over my head, afraid of having poison gas pumped through my central air conditioning. I'm also afraid of fighting. I haven't been in a fistfight since sixth grade. The first sign of trouble and I get real small. It's not because I'm philosophically opposed to fighting. It's because I'm a chicken. I'm afraid of so many things, it scares me just to list them. My family thought I took a risk when I became a newspaper writer instead of a lawyer. That wasn't risky; it was stupid. What would have been risky was becoming a novelist instead of a newspaper writer. I was afraid to do that. I was even afraid to cheat on my wife, and only about a billion husbands cheat on their wives. Nine years married and I didn't stray once, not even a one-nighter, and I was on the road as a sportswriter for eight years; I saw more round heels than Thom McAn. If anyone actually asked me why I was faithful, I said it was because my marriage was too good and my morals too tall, which was, in fact, a partial score. I loved my wife. But also, I was afraid to run around; I wasn't afraid of getting caught as much as I was afraid of risking rejection.

But if I couldn't be fearless in person, I could always be sassy in print. I had work to do, didn't I? And now was as good a time as any to test my editors' advice that relief was available through hard work. Cut the chatter, sweetheart, get me John Calvin.

I began looking through my notes. I'd spent four hours at an accordion competition. I'd done at least twenty interviews. Somewhere in there was a bush onto which I could spray this mood I was in. It didn't take long to find it. It seemed that almost everyone I'd interviewed was Italian, a workable stereotype if I'd ever seen one, and almost all of them had complained that the accordion was maligned as a low-rent musical appliance when it was actually a great classical instrument. Made sense to me. I seemed to recall how Bach wanted to write for accordions, but he was under contract to Steinway, and Steinway said, "Johnny, baby, you're beautiful, kid. You're an artiste, Johnny. Not just an artist, an artiste. But you've gotta stop with this fecockta squeeze-box. You write a couple of catchy tunes for the piano, you're on the charts all over the world. You write for accordion and the only place you'll sell records is Rome. Johnny, baby, we're talking major-league choices here. You wanna be up there with a superstar like Wayne Newton, or you wanna be the opening act for Lou Monti?" I'm sure my editors wanted a straight account of this monumental event, right? So they should have hired Van Cliburn. This is what I gave them:

"Good evening. This is Tom Snyder. The name of the program is 'Tomorrow, Coast-to Coast,' and we're joined in the studio by Mr. Winston Smythe, the world's greatest classical accordionist. Good evening, sir."

"Good evening, Mr. Snyder. Pleasure to be here."

"Thank you, sir. May I call you Carmine?"

"Why?"

"It just seems to fit. Now, Carmine, tell me, which term do classical accordionists prefer for their instrument—the 'Squeeze-box,' or the 'Stomach Steinway'?"

"Actually, we prefer 'accordion.'"

"Then 'accordion' it is, sir. Now, let me ask you a question about classical accordioning—do you use a leash on your monkey?"

"I don't have a monkey. I'm not a street-corner act. I'm a serious musician."

"And a very good one, I'm sure. How about it, Carmine,

Thursday, July 9

would you favor us with a tune? Can you play 'Beer Barrel Polka'?"

"I'd intended on playing a Bach fugue."

"Let's get serious, Carmine. Nobody plays Bach on a squeeze-box. Do 'Lady of Spain.'"

That was the beginning of the piece. After I'd written that and most of the body, I felt a little less hostile, and I called Arthur back. I felt shabby about invoking attorney-client privilege; that was bogus. I shouldn't have done it. Caution is one thing. This was paranoia. First of all, if there's anyone in the family who can help both Karril and me, it's Shelley. Second of all, why was I testing Arthur like that? He and Shelley had the closest relationship of any married couple I knew. All I could accomplish by binding him to secrecy through some ethical technicality was to make him uncomfortable. "I feel lousy about it, Arthur, really. I want you to tell Shelley. I don't know what made me do it. I think this thing is already beginning to make me crazy. Do you understand?"

"I understand," he said soothingly.

"You wouldn't have told her, would you?"

"No, but I'm glad I can now. Because I know how much she loves you; she'll want to help." He hesitated before going on, like a drop of water growing fat on the lip of a faucet. "I sense this is very difficult on you. You sound intimidated, and that's not like you."

I smiled. "Yeah. Right."

"And Karril? Is she nervous too?"

"You'd think so. But actually she's excited. Remember I told you how uneasy I felt about Polly Westin? I wondered if she wasn't just on the point of a very sophisticated sting here? Well, maybe I'm pathologically suspicious, but I mention that to Karril, and she says to me, 'That's your whole makeup.' Like this thing is so clean you can eat off it. I mean, give me a break. I'm afraid Karril wants a kid so bad she'll jump through hoops; all this woman had to do was say the magic word, 'baby,' and Karril put on the blindfold."

"I don't envy your situation."

"It stinks, Arthur. You wait so long for something to happen. Then when it does, the deal has so many holes it's like they wrote it on a mosquito net. Look, I didn't mean to put you in the middle of this. We'll work it out. I just needed some legal advice."

"I'll do everything I can to help. And if you and Karril need any other help, even if you just want moral support, please call us. If you don't call us, we'll call you. We love you, and we want to help; I'm sure Shelley will call you as soon as I tell her about this. And no matter what happens, no matter which way you decide, our prayers are with you."

Whenever Karril worked late I made dinner for us, which was fine because I liked to cook. Tonight's menu was broiled chicken and steamed carrots and pole beans, and I had it timed so I'd get it to the table about five minutes after Karril walked in. It looked great on the plate. I never got to taste it though, because just as we were sitting down, the phone rang.

"Tony, it's Polly. Pick up the extension."

I grabbed some paper and a pen and started upstairs. Halfway up I stopped; I couldn't believe what was happening to me. Sweat was pouring out of me. My forehead. My chin. My thighs. My hands. They were all wet. It was like a water main had burst inside of me. And then I felt my chest tighten, and my heart started thumping. No pain in my teeth, my limbs, or my joints, so it probably wasn't a coronary. But my body seemed about

Thursday, July 9

to explode. I placed my right hand on the middle of my chest and pressed; my heart felt so small and coiled that if I could take it out and tee it up, I'd drive it 250 yards.

I was shocked by what was happening. No doubt I was suffering an anxiety attack, but was Polly Westin's call enough to blast me into it? I'd interviewed movie stars, rock stars, sports stars, United States senators, and nobody got to me like this. Jesus. I'd never even met this woman; I'd only known her name for twenty-four hours. How could she get under my skin like this? I had no choice but to laugh, mostly in nervous admiration. *Morituri te salutamus.* Then I crossed the river from skepticism to contempt. How dare she take control of my life so easily?

I picked up the phone and heard her telling Karril, "Everything's going so well. All the medical tests on the mother are positive. The baby's in excellent health. All signs point to a normal birth, and you ought to be prepared for a large baby, maybe nine or ten pounds."

"Oh, that sounds great," Karril said, more excited than ever.

My turn. "Super," I said. No good. Forced. I wanted sincere, not sarcastic. "We're deeply grateful for what you've done." (I neglected to add, "You bitch.")

"Not at all," Polly said. "Like I said, we're just a group of adoptive parents who want to help others feel the joy we feel." (She neglected to add, "For cash customers.")

But in a way, I believed her. Lots of people get kids this way; she said she got one this way. In her book, *The Baby Brokers,* Lynn McTaggart wrote of Stanley B. Michelman, a New York attorney who, for a considerable fee, arranged private adoptions: "Michelman probably didn't do it strictly for the money. He liked the idea that he was helping desperate women and get-

Thursday, July 9

ting people babies, liked their gratitude, reveled in it, in fact...liked being 'Mr. Stork.'" I saw Polly fitting that description. I couldn't know if she would some day be indicted, tried, and later acquitted for baby brokering as Michelman was, but my guess was she didn't feel she was doing anything wrong. My guess was that on this one Polly Westin stood shoulder to shoulder with Phyllis Schlafly, who once said about this kind of adoption, "Where there's a willing seller and an eager buyer, and the baby moves from an unwanted environment into a home with loving adoptive parents, where's the crime? If there's such a thing as victimless crime, this is it."

I was appalled by the conversation between Polly and Karril. Polly was coming on as more than even a close friend—a cousin, perhaps. She was saying what good times we'd all have together. Her, her husband, her children, us, our adopted baby. Like we were going to timeshare a resort condo together. It was bad enough that she had injected herself into our lives. But now it seemed she wasn't content with the one-shot roller coaster ride around the bloodstream. Now she was acting like she wanted to be surgically bonded to us.

I'd had about enough of this.

"Polly, would it be all right to ask you a few questions?"

"What kind of questions?"

I had to control my tone. I wanted to establish myself as a strong person in her eyes, so she didn't think she could just go through us like crap through a goose, as George Patton used to say. But it was important that my attitude be suppliant, not adversarial. I couldn't play bump-and-run with her just to show her how tough I was. It would be self-defeating. She had the supply; I had the demand; I was a dime a dozen. The situation reminded me of the scene in the movie *Raiders of the*

44

Thursday, July 9

Lost Ark, in which the Arab with the scimitar makes about forty-five twirling, swirling, Middle Eastern kung-fez moves designed to intimidate Indiana Jones, and then Jones calmly takes out his pistol, shrugs, and shoots the bozo. So much for fancy footwork. I had to remember Polly had the pistol.

"About the baby's background?"

"The baby is healthy; I told you that. Both parents are white. There is no history of disease or drug addiction. Look, this is a healthy baby. Don't be so concerned. You two are just so lucky that this is happening, that you have a chance to get this baby."

I was sure Karril was shaking her head, yes, yes, so lucky, yes. "Oh, we are lucky, Polly, and I don't mean to upset you, but we'd just like to know as much as we can about our child." I deliberately said *our child* hoping it would sound good to Polly.

"I'm telling you all I know."

"Well, I ask questions a lot in my line of work, so maybe you could just bear with me. We wondered about the natural parents' background. Are they Irish? Polish? Italian? Greek?" I assumed they weren't Jewish. There probably aren't as many illegitimate Jewish babies born per year as there are solar eclipses. Not only do Jews have no religious taboo against abortion, but studies show that they are a most sophisticated group in terms of effective contraception and family planning.

"I'll try to find out for you. Does it matter?"

"No, not at all." I didn't like the edge in her voice, and I thought I might be pushing too hard. It really didn't matter. I just wanted to know. It may seem terribly narrow-minded, but I wanted some clue to what the baby might look like, and I thought this would help. Is that so awful? I tried to sound cheery. "All that really matters is that everyone's healthy. But if it's no trouble finding out the natural parents' heritage, we'd like to know. The day may come when the child will want to know."

"Right now all I know is that we can assure you that both parents are white and healthy, and that the pregnancy is going along without any complications."

Assure us? I'm supposed to believe that? "How old are the parents?" There might be a health problem with a thirteen- or fourteen-year-old mother.

"I don't know. I'll find out."

"Where are they from?"

"New York."

"State or city?" Ease off. You're not cross-examining a witness. "I only ask that, you know, because we're originally from Queens and Long Island." Weak.

"The city, I believe."

"That's nice." Having gone to college in upstate New York, I was unalterably, if wrong-headedly, convinced that city kids were sharper. The way I handicapped it, a New York City zip code was worth fifteen points on an IQ test. Just by the vibes. "Are they married?"

"No. Why are you asking so many questions?"

What was I supposed to tell her? That I was taking notes? That some of these questions were to satisfy my curiosity, and the others were so I could gather evidence in case I needed it down the line? "I'm sorry. I guess I'm just used to interviewing people."

"This is done through friends. It's done on faith. You have to have faith."

"Sorry. I don't suppose the mother wants to meet us?" I was already thinking ahead to the time I might have to pick her out of a line-up.

"No."

"Do you think it would be possible just to see her, you know, to tell her how much we appreciate this and

Thursday, July 9

how we'll take good care of her baby. I mean, just so she can see we're nice people."

"No. You aren't to see her, and she isn't to see you. You'll never even know her name. The only one who will is her lawyer. You'll never need it. There is to be no contact between you."

That was emphatic. I was backed up by it. "Do we need a lawyer?"

"You'll need one to get the forms straight, and for petitioning the court, and for the naming of the baby when the adoption decree is given. A new birth certificate will be issued with the baby having your last name. I know how it works in Maryland, but I'm not sure about D.C. Get a lawyer, but don't tell him any of the details. You haven't told anyone about this, have you?"

"No. You told us not to."

"Good."

"But wouldn't we want to bring our lawyer with us to pick up the baby?" If she'd said yes to this, Karril could have picked me off the floor with a scraper.

"No. The mother will have her lawyer with her. It's all perfectly legal. Don't worry. You may want to get a pediatrician though, to look at the baby when you bring her home. Yes, call one now, Karril, and make an appointment for the day you bring the baby home."

I was tiring of this thrust and parry. Karril had deferred to me and I was beginning to worry that my monopolization of the conversation wouldn't sit well with Polly. Fact was, we couldn't afford to offend her. She was crucial to the deal, and as long as we went with it, we'd have to work with Polly. So okay, let's get to the big one.

"Polly," I said, "you weren't clear about the money yesterday."

"It's $15,000."

Thursday, July 9

Good God, she was serious. For a second I was dumbstruck. I thought that was just a high-end ballpark figure to see how we were fixed. Fifteen thousand dollars. We had it. I had saved it over eleven years of working. But my God, *I was actually being sold a baby.*

"That's a lot of money," I said rather breathlessly.

"I told you it might cost that much," she said. Not even a hint of softness in her voice anymore.

"But why so much?"

"It isn't so much. People pay up to $50,000 on the Black Market. We paid almost $10,000 for our daughter four years ago. You figure in inflation and $15,000 isn't much at all—if you really want a baby." She was stone cold as she said, "There is to be no negotiation on the fee. The mother has asked for that much, and that's it. I need a fast commitment."

"We've got it," I said.

"I need a definite commitment. Other couples are interested in this baby; they're out there waiting. We went to one couple before you, but they couldn't come up with the money. You're sure you can?"

Money talks, bullshit walks. So what else is new? I could hardly claim to be surprised, but I wondered if Karril had picked her jaw off her lap yet. I had Polly's words from yesterday in front of me: My contact in New Jersey called and asked me if I knew of a couple here who would give the baby a good home and I immediately thought of you.

Sure. Hardball after all. I made my voice into a hammer. "I said, we've got it."

"In cash?"

"In cash."

"Good," Polly said, like we'd just signed a contract. I checked my fingertips for blood. "My contact in New Jersey is named Grace Zimmer; she'll be in touch with you

Thursday, July 9

sometime soon. I want you to call me after she calls you. I want you to call me after each time she calls you, you know, tell me what she says, so if there are any problems or questions we can go over them. And call me after any conversation you have with your lawyer or your pediatrician. Remember to call."

There was about as much snow in Florida as there was trust in this woman. Once more to the notes: This is done through friends. It's done on faith. You have to have faith.

Tell me again about the rabbits, George.

I was smiling just listening to her. She should have been a jukebox the way she could change tunes.

"I really want to meet you both; I'm sure we're going to be such good friends," she said. "Karril, you and I will go out and buy a crib and some furniture and baby clothes together; I know a place where we can get a great discount. I'll help you in whatever way I can. Now don't worry. Everything's going to work out. Just think about becoming parents. Think about going to New York and holding that baby in your arms."

Fifteen thousand dollars. Jesus.

I sat upstairs with my eyes closed imagining dollar bills with wings flying out my bedroom window. One after another. Fifteen thousand George Washingtons, revving up, winking at me, taking off, flying away. So long, sucker.

I couldn't decide which infuriated me more, the immorality of putting a price tag on a baby, or the specific price tag on this baby. This wasn't adoption, it was a purchase. COD. All sales final. And knowing Karril wanted *this* baby more than I did made me even angrier, because I became fastened to the notion that I was buying this baby for her.

Thursday, July 9

  Karril had been brought up to believe that the way marriage worked, the man was the provider. He went out to work and his salary paid for everything. The woman stayed home and cared for the children. If there weren't any children, the woman stayed home and waited for them, presumably the way one waits for a delivery from UPS. If the woman chose to go out and work, whatever money she earned was hers to spend as she pleased. If she wanted to spend it all on herself, that was her prerogative.
  What was his, was hers.
  What was hers, was hers also.
  I didn't like the philosophy. I never approved it. In fact, I did everything I could to dissuade her from it. It was anachronistic, and it clearly put her out of step with the rest of the women of her generation who were marching to the beat of a liberated drummer.
  I graduated from college on a Friday and was working by the next Monday. I was proud of having started at $150 a week and increasing it steadily until now I was earning five times that. I thought that was pretty damned good. But I was prouder still of having been a responsible wage earner and saver. Whatever I bought, I paid for in cash. I owed no one. I earned my own way.
  I understood that Karril hadn't been raised to have any career other than motherhood; I had no gripe with that. But I couldn't understand why she was so reluctant to get a job while she waited for the children. What made her think she was so much better than everyone else that she deserved the privilege of sitting at home and watching soap operas all day? I mean, at what point did they stop waiting around for Amelia Earhart and send the band home?
  I'd say, "Karril, I don't think you ought to stay home anymore. No woman your age who doesn't have kids

Thursday, July 9

just sits around like this. It's terribly destructive. You've got to get up and go to work. You've got to be around people. The more you isolate yourself, the more you bathe in self-pity, the lower your self-esteem will drop and the harder it'll be to break the cycle."

Eventually she would find a job. But always some drone job with no prospect for advancing. Since Karril didn't want to work in the first place, jobs like these extracted no emotional investment. If she got laid-off, it was no big deal. If she quit, there was nothing worth regretting.

Over the years I came to resent the lack of equality in the marriage. It seemed unfair to me that while I was working as hard as I could and being responsible enough to deny myself creature comforts so I could build up a balance in our joint savings account, that Karril was tripping in and out of goofball jobs at her whim, la-di-da, and, I thought, spitting in my eye for suggesting she work at all. I got tired of carrying her; I'm not UNICEF.

Ultimately she came to agree that it was, in fact, unfair. And although she never lost her distaste for work, she stopped vetoing the idea. In our last year on Long Island she got a good sales job at Bloomingdale's, and in Washington she got a good job selling bridal gowns. She voluntarily used her salary to cover our household expenses, put some of what was left into our savings account, and spent the rest, with my sincere blessing, on whatever she wanted. All things being equal, I should have called us even.

But fifteen big ones. You know?

In a few short minutes I'd really worked up a sweat about them. I was so mad that had my teeth been in backwards, I'd have chewed myself to death.

When Karril came up the stairs after the phone call from Polly, I put up my hand like a traffic cop and

Thursday, July 9

announced that what I was about to say I was only going to say once, and I wanted no rebuttal, no argument, not even civilized discussion. "I may be totally wrong about this. It may be the furthest thing from your mind. If so, I apologize in advance. But $15,000 is all we've got. It took me long years of hard work to save it, and I think it's fair to say that it was primarily my work and my years that went into acquiring it. Now, we may get this baby. I hope we do. But Karril, there is no way I can see myself buying you this baby like it's some kind of gift. No way."

I'd drawn a line in the sand.

As I watched the color drain from my wife's face I knew we were on different sides.

She was always articulate with her eyes, and her eyes were calling me names I didn't think she knew. Resentment sprayed from her like buckshot, stinging me up and down.

"I can't believe you," she said.

"I don't want to discuss it. I said it. I meant it. It's over," I said, standing to try and intimidate her into silence.

"How can you say you're buying me a gift?" she asked. She was flustered, stammering from anger. Tears had already formed in her eyes and as they dripped down her cheeks they appeared to steam. "How can you even think that?"

I backed off and sat still.

"It's your money, I know that," she said. "You saved it, I didn't. You can do what you want with it, but don't you dare say that I want you to buy me this baby. This is a baby, not a sewing machine or a coffee table. Tony, I just don't understand you. For years you've been pushing me to adopt; I thought you really wanted a baby. I can't say I appreciate how much money $15,000 is,

Thursday, July 9

except that I can't even imagine how many years it would take me to save that much. But if this is the way it's done, and we want to become parents, then we've *got* to do it. I never thought the money would matter to you. You're always saying you saved it for a family—now we've got the chance to have a family. Why do you think it's for me? Isn't it for us?"

I didn't know. I honestly didn't know.

I was confused. Something else, something other than the money was discomfiting me. It wasn't yet tangible, but it was gathering, I could feel it. I just couldn't identify it.

I looked blankly at Karril. I thought I ought to say something, so I said, "I'm sorry," and reached out for her and brought her close to me and held her and stroked her hair. Even as I was trying to convince myself that we could be in this together, the voice inside my head was saying we were in it alone.

When the phone rings after eleven-thirty at night I automatically assume the worst; at least dismemberment, probably death. Anything else holds until morning.

From the way Karril sat up in bed after answering I knew the caller was Grace Zimmer, so I went downstairs and got on the extension quickly. I immediately felt better about Grace than Polly. I know that's not necessarily saying much; although Caligula killed fewer people than Hitler, you wouldn't want either to give you a haircut. But I liked the balance of Grace's voice. As a reporter, I spent a lot of time on the phone interviewing people, and I respected a professional sound. Polly struck me as having a petty bureaucrat mentality; I fixed Grace much higher on the administrative ladder. She was better informed, more receptive to questions, more consistent.

Thursday, July 9

I had confidence in the information she gave us. And when she cheerfully agreed to get us some additional information we requested I didn't sense any suspicion of our motives, as I had from Polly. My first read on Grace Zimmer was that you could make a deal with her. Not that I'd trust her completely. Blind trust is for the very rich or the very pious.

I desperately wanted a child. I would have done almost anything to have one. But as emotionally vulnerable to the prospect as I was, I wouldn't let myself be emotionally blackmailed into it, and so I saw my relationship to Polly, Grace, and whoever else was involved in this as adversarial. Before I'd let any one of them put that baby in my arms I'd show them how tough and thorough a reporter I was. I got righteous.

I'd be all over their case like water on a frog. And despite my personal, emotional involvement, when it came to gathering facts, I could be so detached you'd think I'd been amputated. From now on, so far as I was concerned, this was strictly business.

There was a baby for sale.

We were sure we wanted one. But did we want *this* one? And did we want this one this *way?*

The sellers had established price as their concern. I didn't know how much, if any play there would be in the number, but as the buyer, my concern was fair value. On this level it was like buying a car, and before I got carried away with the deluxe option package—the sport mirrors; the velour buckets; the mahogany-grained dash—I had to know what came standard, factory equipped.

Most important was the baby's health; I wasn't buying damaged goods.

Grace sought to assure us. "The natural mother has had a normal, healthy pregnancy. An *excellent* preg-

Thursday, July 9

nancy. She's passed every test with flying colors, and believe me, she's had them all."

When someone wants to sell you something, the word "good" isn't good enough. It's always "excellent," or "ideal," or "wonderful," or "perfect." If they think you are a real fish they'll say "very excellent," or "very ideal." That word "very" is crucial. Very crucial. The rule is: accentuate the positive, eliminate the negative. To foster the proper attitude for an adoption the seller should say, "If it was my own daughter I couldn't feel any more comfortable with the situation. *It's very perfect.*" Even though you know that only an idiot would believe this, it makes you happy to hear it because you desperately want to believe that there is no possibility of anything being wrong with this child, that this baby is, indeed, the Gerber baby. Would you consider, even for a moment, the child if the baby seller told you, "The natural mother is a big, fat, dumb sloth who smokes, drinks, and carries on, and who is likely to give birth to something resembling a hippopotamus, and a slow one at that." So I smiled to myself and let Grace keep selling.

"The girl and her foster mother have gone to great lengths to have a perfect pregnancy; they've had an obstetrician for months," Grace said proudly.

Foster mother?

Now there's a red flag.

I made a note and circled it. I'd get back to that later.

"There's nothing I can tell you other than there's nothing in either natural parent's background, healthwise, that you have to worry about," Grace said. She said the identity of the natural father was known, that he and the natural mother had agreed to place the child directly with adoptive parents. "And don't worry," Grace said reassuringly, "if anything's wrong with the baby at birth, the baby will not be put up for adoption."

I breathed a sigh of relief and scratched one question off my list. We wouldn't get stuck with a defective model. If the kid came out of the oven with one arm, or no ears, it was a tough break all around, but at least it wouldn't cost us. I admit my response was so coarse it seemed reptilian. But they'd set the ground rules; I was just trying to play by them.

"And what if later, maybe in a month or two, a genetic problem surfaces?" I asked. Bottom line, I didn't want to get stuck with a baby who'd end up dead or institutionalized; I was looking for some kind of guarantee. If I didn't have to take delivery on a baby with obvious imperfections, why should I have to keep one who starts falling apart after a few spins around the block? Jesus, you wait nine years for a baby and you end up negotiating a leasing agreement.

"I don't know," Grace said. "That never entered into it when we adopted." She was silent for a few seconds. I assumed I had stumped her, and even if it was a stupid game I felt good that I was winning. "I think you might want your own physician to examine the baby in the hospital," she said, as if offering a compromise. "By the way, the baby will be born in Flushing Hospital."

Flushing. A working-class section of Queens. Maybe some clue to the economic and ethnic backgrounds of the parents? Another something to get back to.

"Can we do that?" I asked. "I mean, get our own physician to examine the baby in the hospital?"

"Of course. Look, you don't have to take this baby if you don't want to. A lot of times adoptive parents choose not to, even at the last minute. We want you to be perfectly happy with your baby."

That was a very perfect thing to say.

Grace was good. I had the round-by-round even to that point.

Thursday, July 9

"What about the lawyers?" I asked.

"The foster mother already has a lawyer. All the papers have already been drawn up. It's illegal to have the natural mother sign the consent forms before she delivers, but after she delivers she'll sign them."

"Then this is legal?"

"Oh yes."

"And can you give us the name of her lawyer?" I wanted to check out his background. I had him figured for a dirtball who'd take down a big chunk of the $15,000 himself. If I got lucky I could expose him in print and get him disbarred. If I got very lucky I could persuade him to make restitution, then expose him in print and get him disbarred. Just because I'm ethical doesn't mean I'm not vindictive.

"I don't have the name now. I'll get it."

"You see, Grace, what we're really worried about is that years from now we'll get this knock on our door, and it'll be the natural mother, coming with a court order to claim her kid."

"That won't happen. There is no chance of this girl changing her mind. She wants to give up the baby and go on with her life. A social worker has been assigned to her case, and they've been working together."

A social worker?

My eyes lit up. Was it possible that a duly accredited and licensed employee of the City of New York was in on this too, and had cut herself a slice of my pie? Catching a lawyer with his hands dirty is good, but catching a civil servant *in bribo flagranto,* as they say, is very excellent. Hold Page One. As Grace continued speaking, I wrote down "social worker" and circled it. Another name I'd need.

"The girl has been positive about direct adoption all along," Grace said. "She doesn't even want to know what sex the baby is. She's told her doctor to knock her out just before she gives birth, and not to tell her anything about the baby. She can't even find out where the baby's going. Only the lawyer, the social worker, and the foster mother will know. And the papers will be sealed by the court."

"But we have no guarantee," I said imploringly.

"Believe me, the girl has no recourse because of the consent forms she's signing."

I let it rest. Better not to tell her that I'd spoken to a lawyer and I believed that the money made it illegal—made it coercion—and even if the natural mother was party to an illegal act, she could still petition the court to get her baby back. Better not to antagonize Grace. I had precious little control as it was. If we had to lose this baby, I wanted it to be because we made the call. Not Grace Zimmer.

"I'm a little concerned about the money. I have it. But can't I give you some by check?"

"No. It has to be cash. Nothing is to be traceable."

I let the apparent contradiction between "oh yes, it's legal" and "nothing is to be traceable" pass. And as innocently as possible under the circumstances I said, "I understand. Where will the money go?"

"To the girl ultimately, to finish her college education."

Nice touch. I didn't believe even a syllable, but I admired the forethought of the answer.

"She's in college?"

"They both are. This baby came along at a bad time for them. She might have had an abortion, but it was already too late when she found out she was pregnant. She just wants to go on with her life."

"An abortion? Then she's not Catholic?"

Thursday, July 9

"I don't know. I can find out if you want. I know she's not Jewish. Is it important?"

"No, but I'd like to find out. I mean, if it's not any trouble."

"I'll find out. Now, what else would you like to know?"

"How old is she?"

"She's nineteen. So is the boy."

Good. Not one of the fifteen-year-old teenyboppers at the Burger King getting popped in the back seat of a Camaro.

"You mentioned a foster mother. Is there any trouble in the girl's family? Is she a runaway?" I wasn't at all comfortable with the notion that the mother of my child was some overripe street plum.

"No. She grew up in Woodside. There was some confusion in the girl's family years ago, a financial problem I think, and she left to live with the foster mother as a teenager. She's not there now; she's on her own. She has a perfectly wonderful relationship with her parents now, but she feels closer to the foster mother, and the foster mother helped her through this."

Although Grace's explanation was reassuring, I remained troubled by the circumstances. My middle name is Overreact, and Woodside being one step down from Flushing, my conclusion was that this was a poor girl from a broken home who was unquestionably a delinquent and possibly a felon. I heard my father's voice in my head, warning me about the bad seed. All I had to be told now was that she rooted truffles.

"Was the girl *remanded* to the foster mother by the court?" I asked, as if I was auditioning for Perry Mason.

"I don't know. Maybe," Grace said, almost defensively. Then, quickly, she became territorial, jumping in

59

my face. "What difference does it make? She's a perfectly fine girl, and all you should care about is that she's about to give birth to a perfectly healthy baby."

"I guess you're right." I didn't have to marry the girl—just be her baby's father. "I just worry."

"Well, don't worry. I can assure you that the girl is just lovely."

"Have you met her?"

"No, but I've talked with her on the phone, and she sounds lovely. And I've met the foster mother. I sat with her and got the health backgrounds on the girl and the boy. Believe me, this woman is a saint. You couldn't ask for a better home situation than hers. She and her husband just bought a new house in Bayside, and two nicer people you wouldn't want to meet."

"Do they run a foster-care home?" If played right, a professional foster-care home was a big bucks deal. People who do it would know the baby-sale market well enough to set the number at fifteen.

"Not at all. This is a special situation. The foster mother and the girl just happened to hit it off."

I figured I had no shot at this, but there wouldn't be any harm in trying, so I asked, "Grace, would it be possible for us to get the name of the foster mother?"

"It's Amalfitano," Gloria said. Then she spelled it for me. "A-M-A-L-F-I-T-A-N-O. Judy Amalfitano. Wonderful woman. You know, we actually met a year ago at the bar mitzvah of the son of a mutual friend. I remembered it. I met her and right away fell in love with her."

Amalfitano. Now there were three names: Amalfitano, Zimmer, and Westin. I had to go to the public records and check out all three. Find their husbands' names and check them too. Check for police records.

Thursday, July 9

For yellow sheets. For priors. Check to see if anyone's dirty. I doubted it.

I still burned with the rage of the avenging angel, but I felt it blending with the romance of the private eye. I began seeing myself in a Burberry trenchcoat, slipping in and out of alleys, as silent as a fog. Maybe I could get an address on Amalfitano and go up and confront her. Knock on the door of her nice new house and say, "Hi, I'm the guy who's here to buy the baby." I almost felt as if part of that house would belong to me anyway, since it was my $15,000 that was buying the furnishings. And that thought led to this one: they'd get their $15,000. They'd get it in thousand-dollar bills with sequential serial numbers so they'd be easy to trace and hard to cash. Judy Amalfitano couldn't dare put them in the bank, and she wouldn't dare bring them to Safeway and pay for milk and bread with a crisp new thousand-dollar bill.

That kind of big-timing attracts attention.

People remember.

Friday, July 10

It wasn't yet dawn and I couldn't quite focus clearly, but I didn't need 20/20 vision to see that was a limousine idling gently in the street right in front of my house. It was one of those pearl-gray Cadillacs, so long and cool that you don't want to drive it as much as just sip it for a while.

I heard what sounded like hurried footsteps moving away from me, and as I turned in their direction, I saw her—already down the walk and opening the back door of the limo. She was tall and lithe, and she wore a hooded lace dress that covered her so completely and was so gauzily thin and bone white that for a second I thought she was wrapped in bandages, a ghost floating through the receding purple mist.

I saw her face only in profile, only through tinted windows and only for an instant as the limo pulled away. But what a haunting face it was. Her eyes were crystals; her nose straight and proud; her chin strong; her skin like poured cream, unruffled, unmarked, and so pure as to have been kept under glass. The few curls of hair escaping under her hood were light, either sandy or cane, and as she went by I saw her smile. Even behind the dusky windows her teeth sparkled like buffed ivory.

I was so captivated by her face that the limousine was almost out of sight before I thought to search out its

Friday, July 10

license plate. By then I could still distinguish the DPL insignia but none of the numbers. The flags on the hood identified it as a foreign embassy's car, but it was too dark to pick out the colors, and I was left with my guesses. Maybe she was royalty; at least on a diplomatic mission. But what? And why here? Why was she running from my house?

My curiosity overwhelmed my fear, and as I stepped outside I saw it sitting there on the top step—one of those fancy wooden picnic baskets with the hinges in the middle so either end opens. I felt sure she left it for me, and I reached for it. My right hand was no more than an inch from the handles when I heard the soft gurgle coming from within, and I felt myself tremble at realizing that something was alive inside there. I bent down to the end where the sound was and pulled the flap back gently, as if turning the page of a rare, old manuscript. My God, it was a baby. Left on my doorstep. A living, breathing, beautiful baby.

I looked up furtively to see if anyone was looking at me—if there were cameramen, or policemen, or whoever else was supposed to come leaping out of the bushes at me at such a preposterous moment. Nothing. No one. Just me and this baby, gurgling and smiling up at me. Then I saw the note, folded over with my name delicately lettered on the front. I opened it. I was shaking so that I feared I might come apart in sections. "Mr. Tony Kornheiser, I am a big fan of yours. I can tell from the way you write that you will make a wonderful father. Please love my baby."

Imagine, a baby left for me just because someone liked my writing. And all these years I was willing to settle for a nice letter to the editor.

I suppose you want to know if it was a boy or a girl. So do I.

Friday, July 10

I was just about to pick the baby up and find out, when the telephone rang, waking me up, stopping my dream.

Grace.

At seven-thirty in the morning. True to her word, she had the name of the lawyer who was drawing up the adoption papers; she must have called Amalfitano right after hanging up with us at midnight.

W. Allan Cavas, of Richmond Hill.

"You'd better speak to a lawyer in Washington to see if you need any more forms than the standard adoption consent," Grace said. "When you get a lawyer, have him call Mr. Cavas and give Mrs. Amalfitano's name as a reference. Remember now, Mrs. Amalfitano is paying Mr. Cavas's fee, and he is only arranging consent papers—he is not aware of any other transactions." She paused, as if invoking the covenant of conspiracy, then cautioned, "Neither should your lawyer be."

I let it pass. To go along is to play along.

Grace moved ahead to the plan for transferring the baby. Although Polly claimed to need an immediate commitment, there was, in fact, no real urgency. Apparently the birth wasn't imminent, and in any event we wouldn't be given the baby until after its release from the hospital, which Grace figured for four days after its birth. Then, Karril and I—"or an agent in your place," Grace said—would bring the money to Grace's home in Clifton, New Jersey and exchange it for the baby and the adoption forms. After the transfer Grace would take the money to Mrs. Amalfitano at a prearranged site, somewhere between Clifton and Bayside, and that would be that; there would be no need for any of us to see each other again. Obviously, if we could use an agent, there was no need for any of us to see each other at all.

Friday, July 10

At first it struck me as quite naïve of them to allow someone other than us to actually take possession of the baby, but quickly I realized it was I who was being naïve; what mattered most to the sellers wasn't our goodwill, but our hard cash.

Again I did nothing to create distrust in Grace's mind. I simply said, "Fine. I understand."

"Did I tell you about the sonogram?" Grace asked.

"No," Karril said. "The girl had a sonogram?"

"Yes, about a week ago, and everything was excellent."

I didn't know a sonogram from a telegram, but essentially it is a picture of the baby in the womb. Doctors use sonograms to make sure the baby is positioned correctly. In some cases it is possible to determine the sex of the child from the sonogram, and it was Karril's suspicion that this was known but was being deliberately withheld from us. Karril based her suspicion on Polly's occasional reference to the baby as "she," although she conceded that since Polly had a daughter, it would be natural for her to use the pronoun "she" when referring to any child.

Part of my job description is a healthy sense of suspicion, but even if Karril was correct I could appreciate their reluctance to tell us the baby's sex before the birth; they might fear us backing out of the deal if the sex wasn't the one we wanted. What they couldn't possibly know, however, was that Karril wanted a girl, and I wanted a boy. In any case, Grace didn't suggest what color booties to buy, and we didn't ask.

"By the way," Grace said, "the girl has an appointment with her doctor on July 13. If she hasn't delivered by then, she may be induced."

I hoped not. At least not on that day.

65

Friday, July 10

"You had some questions last night," Grace said.

"Yeah," I said. "About medical problems."

"I spoke with Mrs. Amalfitano about that. She agreed to take the baby back if any latent birth defect surfaced after you brought the baby home. She also said if that happened, some of the money would be returned."

It seemed like a good faith gesture on their part, and not wanting to upset the delicate balance I didn't ask how much.

"Was there another question?" Grace asked.

"The mother's ethnic background," I said. It honestly didn't matter. I just wanted to *know*.

"The girl is Irish, Italian, and German, and the boy is Irish."

"Fine. Great," I said.

"I spoke with the girl last night," Grace said, as if about to unwrap a present. "She was bright and bubbly and quite forthright. She hoped the baby would be raised with some religious training, but she had no preference which religion."

"Great. No problem." I was reacting so enthusiastically to these bones of information that I must have seemed like a slobbering dog.

"By the way, she asked about you both. I told her how nice you are. And she said to thank you for wanting her baby and giving it a good home."

I don't know why Grace chose to say that. Whether it was kindness, or manipulation—or a combination of both. I only knew that at that moment she had turned the screws too tight, and I began picking splinters from my heart.

When we got off the phone Karril was smiling. It was her teenager smile, one I'd often seen years ago but hardly at all lately. It jolted me back to the time we'd met, thirteen years earlier at summer camp, before the

Friday, July 10

colitis, before the infertility, before the nasty, surreptitious war of nerves between us. Back to when we were innocent and optimistic, when our futures were blank canvases, and life was an artist with only pastels on the palette. I'd fallen in love with a sunny girl only to watch her set into a murky woman. Seeing that old smile made me shiver to think how much I'd missed it.

"Irish. Got a shot at green eyes and red hair," Karril said, twinkling. "You know how you feel about green eyes and red hair."

I blushed; I surely did favor green eyes and red hair. "How do you think the name Brendan Kevin Sean Patrick Kornheiser will go over when we enroll him in Hebrew School? Instead of chanting prayers at his bar mitzvah this kid will probably recite Yeats. Hey, bet you a dollar we want him to be a lawyer, and he wants to be a cop."

"And what if he's a she?"

A she?

It had never occurred to me that he could be a *she*. In all my many musings about what my child might be like I can honestly say it was always a he—a son, about 6–1, 185; my boy Bill is as straight and as tall as a tree, is he.

I had a fix on him as an infant: I'd be changing his diapers one afternoon; he'd look up at me, wink, then shoot a stream of pee right in my eye—just so I couldn't get overconfident. I had a fix on him as a teenager: we'd be going one-on-one in the driveway. He'd take it to the hoop and I'd summon all the strength left in my old, aching legs and go up with him, swat his shot into the rhododendrons and shout, "In your face disgrace." And I had a fix on him as a young adult: he'd be the only white player in the NBA, and after leading his team to the league championship he'd tell the national television

Friday, July 10

audience that all the credit for his phenomenal shooting should go to his father, the former second team All-Intramural point guard from Harpur College, who always told him, "You're a white boy, so you'll never leap. But if you've got a quick release, and you can stick it from twenty-two feet, you can play with anybody."
    A she? How could I teach a she to pick and roll?
    For a second I was dumbstruck.
    But only for a second.
    "The way I see it," I told Karril, "we have two options. We can trade her to the gypsies in return for a roof job. Or, we can name her Golda Kathleen, buy her a lifetime supply of emery boards and designer jeans and thank God for the money we'll save on the nose job."
    We both laughed and got dressed for work.

    I am a writer by choice, but a reporter by trade. Not an investigative reporter. Those guys are the samurai of the profession, the righteous killers, the superstars. We feature writers are journalism's tap dancers, its window dressing. At our roughest maybe we bruise a few egos. They're in the combat zone; we're in the chorus line.
    I have long nurtured a deep, abiding envy of top investigative reporters. True confessions: when working for the *New York Times* I daydreamed that Seymour Hersh would ask me to join him on investigative projects. Here at the *Washington Post* I've had similar daydreams about teaming up with Bob Woodward, a sort of velvet and steel pas de deux. I covet their status as well as their talent. But after eleven years in this trade even a stylist learns how to follow a trail. Give me a story I care about and put a phone in my hand, and the fact is, I can *play*.

Friday, July 10

The baby sellers had what I wanted; I wanted the kid, and I wanted a story. I didn't think they had to be mutually exclusive. Sitting at my desk at work, running my fingers eagerly over the touch-tone phone I used as a bazooka, I knew the chase was on, and it felt positively invigorating.

My first call was to my father, to update him. He'd adjusted rather well to the prospect of adoption. In fact he was almost enthusiastic about it. It seems that his cursory survey of the condo revealed many grandchildren via the adoption route, so there was no stigma as far as he was concerned. But he was still wary of the legality of the payment. As was I.

Call number two was to the New York City money fund where we had most of our savings. I had a telephone redemption account, and I told the customer service representative to transfer fifteen-thousand dollars to my local savings account at the Riggs Bank in Washington. I was assured that Riggs would have the cash on hand Monday morning. That was time enough since even if the baby was born today, it would not leave the hospital until Monday at the earliest.

The last of the table-setting calls was to my cousin, Arthur. He had spoken to a Florida adoption specialist who was concerned about such a high price for a baby. The inherent risk of a court voiding the consent could not be ignored, so he couldn't advise going ahead. But Arthur again said people have taken it. It depended on how badly they wanted a baby. He said the court rarely saw its function as an investigator. If a solid bond between parent and adopted child has been formed the court was unlikely to decide that the best interests of the child required removing it from a healthy, loving home and remanding it to a single parent who may have

Friday, July 10

already cast considerable doubt as to her fitness.

The most important thing, he said, was to make sure the paperwork was in order so the legal process could function routinely; it was imperative to have a proper release in hand before transporting the child from New Jersey, across state lines, to the District of Columbia. You wouldn't want to violate any interstate compact. In closing, he said he would try and get information about adopting in Florida, and he sent love from my cousin Shelley.

I decided to hold off researching Polly Westin and Grace Zimmer for the moment, figuring they were small change compared to Judy Amalfitano and her lawyer, W. Allan Cavas. I wanted an address and a phone number on Amalfitano in case I wanted to drop by and say hi. But I didn't know her husband's name, and the information operator told me there were more than fifteen Amalfitanos listed in Queens, and eight more unlisted. So Amalfitano went on hold.

I checked out W. Allan Cavas in *Martindale-Hubbell*, the reference guide to lawyers. He'd graduated from Southampton College on Long Island and Portland State law school in Oregon. Portland State from Long Island? Any further west and he gets wet. What was his safe school, Tokyo State? And he was in private practice in the Richmond Hill section of Queens. Admittedly it was a snobby judgment I was making, but I pegged him as a lightweight. It wasn't Harvard and Yale, and it wasn't a big firm in Manhattan. My guess was he worked out of a storefront near Amalfitano's neighborhood, and she'd hired him because he was close by. Maybe he'd done her real estate deal.

I called the New York State Bar Association and found out W. Allan Cavas had been admitted to the bar in

Friday, July 10

1972 and was a member in good standing. There hadn't been any judgments against him. I considered the possibility that he was straight, not wired into this fix. But if he wasn't, the day would come when he'd read about himself in his morning paper and it would be goodbye license.

Next I went to Richard Cohen, who writes a column at the *Post,* ostensibly because Polly Westin had once told Mona—the woman who worked with Karril and was our initial contact—that she knew Cohen. I hoped he could place her and give me some sense of what she was about. But I wanted Cohen's advice even if he didn't remember her, which he didn't. I liked Cohen. I liked his writing and his values. Unlike so many columnists who need to speak for the people, Cohen spoke *to* the people. He didn't write about the Kurd War, or the middle-class coalition the Democrats needed to forge to win control of the school boards in Iowa. He was smart, and he could be sarcastic, but his ideology seemed to be that life was a series of moral choices, and most of the time you didn't have to be Spinoza to pick right from wrong. I liked to think that Cohen and I were kindred spirits, two New Yorkers cast into that vast wilderness beyond the Hudson to bring common sense (and maybe the egg cream) to the philistines. I liked to think that if I had a column I'd write mine the way Cohen wrote his.

We often schmoozed, and typically when we did my end of the conversation sounded like material for a comedy showcase in the Catskills. This being no exception I started out with a brief sketch of the adoption deal, then did some shtick: "Everybody and his brother is having babies except me and Ling Ling. You think it's fun wondering who's going to be the last one left on Earth without a kid, you or a panda? I need this aggra-

Friday, July 10

vation, right? I know fags who have more kids than me. The welfare rolls are top-heavy with women who pop babies out like toast. We're trying nine years. Zippo. We make the Sahara look fertile. Maybe we're doing it wrong. I knew it was a mistake to send away for that do-it-yourself sex manual from Taiwan. And now we get a deal like this.

"These baby sellers, they've got files a mile wide. You want an athlete? They've got the product of two college students in California who jog thirty-five miles a day before breakfast; they did it under the stands between events in the decathlon. You want smart? They've got a pregnant girl in Pittsburgh who plans on getting her doctorate in clinical psychology someday; right now she's fifteen and if she gets tutoring maybe she'll remember when they fought the War of 1812. You want musical ability? They've got a girl in Dallas whose baby was conceived backstage during an Elton John concert. You get what you pay for, right?

"For fifteen grand they put you behind the wheel of a brand new, healthy, bouncy baby. Fifteen grand a little steep, pal? For eight grand you can probably get a slightly used two-year-old; don't worry, it comes with a new baby warranty. For three grand you can leave the showroom with a no-frills kid. Okay, he's only got one ear, but maybe he'll grow up to be a great painter. I mean it's just like buying a Plymouth. I like this baby, yeah, but I'm looking for something with better gas mileage. And it's definitely got to come with FM stereo. By the way, you got anything with chrome? I've always been crazy about chrome."

After I got the sarcasm out of my system Cohen and I had a serious talk. It turned out he had written a couple of stories in 1975 about Bobby Burns, then a Miami Beach lawyer, who ran what was literally a baby farm.

Friday, July 10

He took in unwed mothers, fed them, housed them, and paid for their medical care during their pregnancies. After they gave birth he placed the babies with adoptive parents. Burns passed along his costs to the adoptive parents and charged them a fee for his service. It was a turnkey operation; he was his own cottage industry. And in Florida, where there was no limit on adoption fees, it was legal, though it would not have been so in Washington, D.C. Cohen thought the sugar shack setup bizarre. But he said Burns could make a reasonably persuasive moral argument that the best interests of the child were served by adoption into a loving, two-parent home, and that the money was a separate, insignificant issue.

"If you're going to get involved in an adoption like that, even if you're only considering it now," Cohen said, "you have to talk to a lawyer." He suggested I call Sidney Sachs, in town. "He's not only a great lawyer," Cohen said, "but if he can't help you, he'll set it up so you get the best possible person who can."

One for my side.

I called Sachs, mentioned Cohen's name, and was assured by his associate, Sherry Bindeman, that Sachs would get back to me on Monday; he was away for the weekend.

I wanted Sachs because of Cohen's unequivocal recommendation. But I was hot to trot now; I needed a quick fix. So I called the *Post*'s in-house counsel, Bo Jones, whom I sometimes played softball with on Sunday mornings. Without disclosing the particulars I asked for the names of a few Washington lawyers who might be able to explain the local adoption laws. I called one. But she couldn't see me this afternoon, and she put me onto another, Deborah Luxenberg.

I called her and anxiously outlined the terms of the adoption, making sure to elicit client confidentiality be-

Friday, July 10

fore revealing the $15,000 price tag. It didn't particularly bother me when Luxenberg said, "If there is any money paid, it is totally illegal, and I wouldn't be willing to become involved under those circumstances." Since I intended to hold on for Sachs, I didn't need her as a lawyer; I assured her that all I wanted from her was legal interpretation, not representation. I was so persistent that Luxenberg said I "sounded almost desperate." Responding primarily to my emotional state, she agreed to research the laws further and tell me how a direct placement adoption could be legally effected in the District. Her fee would be sixty dollars.

I made a note to call Karril's younger cousin, Fern, a doctor. She was home in Queens, on vacation, after interning in Maine for three years. I wanted her to go to Flushing Hospital and examine this baby as soon as possible after its birth; I wanted someone I trusted giving us a thorough evaluation of the health of the baby. And, looking for every edge we could get, I hoped her medical credentials might allow her to ascertain the name of the natural mother. Maybe she could even go in and talk with her.

I was in my element now, working the phone, gathering facts, planning a strategy. It felt better the more I drifted away from a personal and toward a professional relationship with the story. This was stage one, once again plugging into a reliable reporting technique. As I wrapped myself in the familiar cloth I saw myself less the victim and more the aggressor. But I was still grounded in reality; even as I sought to convince myself that this wasn't my adoption, this wasn't my baby, these slight denials were just to help me function smoothly, nothing more than a mild dose of psychological Valium.

Friday, July 10

And then, with my heart pounding and my adrenaline pumping and my mind-set in the lock-and-load position, I called my closest friends to enlist their help in what would surely become a firestorm if and when it ignited. I called Ted Beitchman, then an editor at *Inside Sports* magazine, and Dan Lauck, a producer at CBS Sports and a former colleague at the *Post*. I knew they wouldn't fail me because journalists are always up for two things—a juicy conspiracy, and a chance to nail the bad guys.

I poured out my story at breakneck speed, and if it wasn't evident to me, it had to be evident to them that I had careened past stage one and had arrived, breathlessly, at stage two, "Ellery Queen." Crossed the line from fact to fantasy, from reality to romance; this wasn't Valium now, it was methamphetamine, and I was snorting.

I started with the assumption that the baby sellers were amateurs. Would a veteran profiteer sell hot goods to a newspaper reporter, especially one from the *Washington Post*, the paper that brought you Watergate? That would be like a drug smuggler knowingly offering a piece of the action to a uniformed cop. Such an act of rank stupidity meant these jokers were beatable, so eminently beatable that if I planned my moves well I might be able to walk out clean with the kid, without paying them one dime.

I needed a master plan. And I needed it soon. All it would take was some thought, and I knew I could think. Like most New York sixties kids, I could think fast. Unfortunately, my method of thinking is rather unconventional. I'm not only New York and sixties, I'm Jewish and verbal. I think out loud. And I never know what I'm thinking until I hear the thoughts come out of my mouth as words. And then, as they tumble out like bushels of tomatoes, I throw away the rotten ones and keep the ripe ones. On a good day my ratio is about four to one. So, I began raving, creating strategy on the dead run, in the hope that a reasonable percentage of it would be viable. I'd already decided to mark the bills. But if I tried to snatch the kid and bolt, I'd need troop support. I guess my initial thoughts were influenced by heavy paranoia because they emerged full-blown like scenes from a Charles Bronson movie. But to me they sounded dead solid sane. Lauck and Beitchman would have to come to the exchange site in separate cars and station themselves at opposite ends of Grace's street. That would give me the option of switching from my car into one of theirs, and allowed each of them to seal off the primary exit route of any possible chase car; we'd get a substantial head start and we'd be hi-balling it down the New Jersey Turnpike like James Dean and Natalie Wood in a car Grace couldn't identify.

And then, on second thought, the Grab Option presented an enormous risk: before we made a run for it we'd have to secure the proper consent forms. There was no way Grace would be dumb enough to hand over the kid and the papers before we handed over the money. So if we flat seized the kid, it was open and shut kidnapping, and when we pulled up to our house in Washington the welcoming committee would be cops bearing cuffs. Even in my wildest fantasy—taking the kid to parts unknown and managing a complete change of identity—without the papers we'd never get a legal adoption. So clearly there was no percentage in stealing the kid.

Then the question became—how much money do we pay? I understood them insisting on cash; a cancelled check would be a weapon in my hands. But could I bargain with them? Would they go for part now and

Friday, July 10

the remainder after the adoption was finalized? Could I intimidate them? Would a threat to expose all the grimy details in print persuade them to lower the price?

It seemed no matter where I turned my wheels, all I succeeded in doing was spinning them. When you got down to it, the Finesse Option was a long shot. Unless I scared the hell out of them they didn't have to bend an inch. Holding that baby was like being dealt a natural royal flush. What's more, they had potential threats of their own. How could I be sure that $15,000 wasn't just the ante? What if they exercised the Extortion Option? How tough would it be for them to threaten to claim coercion and void the adoption unless we came up with some additional money? More scratch for the itch, as it were. They could squeeze us dry on the installment plan.

I knew Beitchman and Lauck would help wherever possible. But the more animated I became, the more I sensed myself babbling, and I lowered my volume. Instead of planning for a kamikaze attack, I settled for self-protection; I'd always looked better in tweed than fatigues anyway. Any new father would be expected to bring a camera when he picked up his kid, so getting pictures of the sellers would be easy. I could also be wired for sound at the transfer by concealing a tape recorder in my jacket pocket. That would give me enough evidence for an audio-visual presentation to a grand jury. Through a contact he had in the FBI Lauck would be able to get Amalfitano's address, and he agreed to go there and check out her and the natural mother. He'd need a ruse to gain entry, but knowing that Amalfitano had just bought a house and was refurbishing it, he could pose as an aluminum siding salesman and no one would question it. Beitchman had relatives in Clifton, and he'd try and get background on the Zimmers through them. He'd also cruise Clifton to get a line on logical sites where Grace and Amalfitano might meet after the transfer so we could attempt to photograph the exchange of money. I wanted him to draw a map of the streets surrounding Grace's house in case we had to pull the Block and Scoot Maneuver because the sellers tried to take the cash and welch on the kid and the papers.

And then the white light of reality hit me. Two could play this game. What if they really tried to screw us? What began as a fantasy escalated rapidly into cold, paranoid terror:

I heard myself asking out loud: "Should I get a gun?"

I wondered if somewhere in Clifton, Grace wasn't asking herself the same thing. If I thought of guns, why shouldn't she?

And if guns were a consideration, what the hell had I gotten myself into?

I called Karril and told her everything that had happened so far, including my contemplation of the gun.

"Guns?" she asked incredulously. "Tony, you're acting crazy."

I hoped I was just acting.

It was getting too thick; I had to get outside myself for a while. Luckily today was Friday, and on Friday I played softball. I pitched in the D.C. Recreation League for Bialystock & Bloom, a team named after Zero Mostel's and Gene Wilder's characters in the movie *The Producers*. Our team consistently won 80 percent of its games. But even if we never scored a run I'd be there each week, on the banks of the Potomac, between the shadows of the Washington and Lincoln memorials. Long ago I learned that the next best thing to winning, was losing. Just getting in the game was therapeutic. I found that the only way I could get my worries off my mind was to put my mind on hold, and the only way I could

Friday, July 10

do that was through physical activity. All I cared about at softball, was softball. So thank God for softball. And thank God for the routine I followed each morning—stretching, one hundred push-ups, one hundred sit-ups—even if these last few days the anxiety pains in my chest were so sharp that I sometimes prayed to black out, if only to be momentarily free from those baby-selling harpies.

We won, and I went home exhausted and happy. But as soon as I walked through the door I threw off that personality as if it were a sweatband, and picked up one marked Manipulative Doomsayer. Conducting what amounted to a filibuster, I painted as bleak a picture of this adoption as possible in an attempt to balance what I saw as my wife's irrational euphoria. The coldness and negativity wrung all the joy from her smile and left the drops in a puddle by her feet. I am sorry for that now, but at the time I thought the only way was to play it, was to play it hard. Paranoia makes fools of us all.

When Karril finally spoke, it was in disgust. "Polly called," she said. By the look on her face I knew the call had been no less pleasant than my entrance.

"And?" I asked.

"And she was very upset that we didn't call her after Grace called us."

"So you told her we didn't get off the phone with Grace until after midnight."

"She didn't care. She said she told us to call her as soon as we had any contact with Grace. She was very upset. Tony, I don't think we can afford to make her angry with us."

I got hot so quick that if I'd been a colt I'd have qualified for the Kentucky Derby. "What is this? A police state? Is this woman going to make these implicit threats every time we don't dot the 'i' or cross the 't'? She doesn't have any papers on us. She's brokering a goddamn baby, and she's probably taking her goddamn cut. Screw her."

"She wants to meet us."

"That figures."

"I think she has to approve us before we get the baby. Obviously, she's working closely with Grace."

"Charlemagne's eyes and ears. Okay, let's set up a time. I don't want her here. Can we go to her house?"

"No. She insists on coming here."

"Can't say that I blame her. I'll try and fit it into my schedule." I had cooled down. Suddenly I got hot again. "You know I don't like this. And I don't like her. I'm not some goddamn criminal coming up for parole."

"She keeps talking to me about going to Crib N' Cradle with her, just to shop around. Price a crib. Price baby furniture. And she insists we buy a car seat to take the baby home. I don't think we ought to buy anything until we decide whether or not we're going through with the adoption."

"I agree with you."

Karril got me in her sights and held me there with her gaze. "Have you made a decision yet?" she asked.

"No," I said. The hole in the conversation widened until it seemed to surround us, and it occurred to me that I should explain myself. "I think we ought to go on like we're going. We're working on getting a lawyer; we're working on checking these people; I'm going to call Fern to examine the baby. We've got time. We don't have to make a decision until we hold the baby in our arms, right?"

"I don't want to wait for that. They put that baby in my arms and I won't want to give it back. That would kill me."

Friday, July 10

"I just don't think we should panic."

"I didn't ask you to panic, Tony. I asked you about a decision."

"I'm no good at decisions. You know that. Half the time I can't even decide what I want for dinner."

"This isn't a dinner; it's a *baby*."

Saturday, July 11

Fern wasn't licensed in New York, and therefore had no hospital privileges at Flushing. Nor did she know any pediatricians who had.

It was going to be left to me to get us a doctor.

By the time I awoke Karril had already gone to work, which was just as well considering the mood I was in. My level of frustration stood so tall I needed a ladder to reach it. The pressure of this adoption was turning me into a madman; I knew that if Karril had been home I'd have picked a fight. Left alone I began pacing through the house, picking up speed as the morning wore on, questioning life and luck in general, and my marriage and "my child" in particular.

Like every other married couple, we'd had good times and bad. On balance, the good far outweighed the bad. We had, after all, stayed together for more than nine years. But it was obvious that these were especially bad times, and the marriage was teetering under the strain. Karril and I were no warmer to each other than two bags of dry ice doing the minuet.

Still, I thought we would survive it. We'd survived bad times before. I loved Karril very much. I cleaved to her for those specific qualities she had which I didn't: kindness; softness; trust; a lack of duplicity. She filled in my blanks. Over the years, primarily because of her

Saturday, July 11

physical fragility, the nature of our relationship had shifted to where she often needed protection more than passion, and we were concerned more with immunization against pain than the pursuit of pleasure. But there was no need to assign blame for what had evolved. On some acceptable level we were satisfying our psychic needs. We'd both worked diligently, if not wisely, at cultivating this dependency, and our styles—my aggressiveness, her passivity—nurtured it. The good news about wearing a thick lead shield is that it protects you from invasive X-rays; the bad news is that very quickly you stagger with the weight.

Confronting my true feelings about adopting was more disturbing. I had pushed Karril toward adopting, and now I was backing away. I'd been hammering away at the questionable legality of this adoption. Although, in truth, I suspected the chances of getting burned were slim, I created the impression that they loomed so large as to blot out the sun. But that was just a pose, a defense mechanism. Alone now, I couldn't avoid the inquiry into how much I really wanted this baby. Which was—not much. It hadn't felt right from the start. The money, the illegality, the bizarre circumstances, those were easy outs. But superficial ones. The whole truth, and nothing but the truth, was that I didn't really want to adopt. Not yet. And not this way.

In 1978, after six years of marriage and four years of trying, and failing, to have children, I concluded we were up against a wall. Having been unable to bust through it, I stepped back, read what seemed to be the writing on it, and made a big push for us to adopt. At first Karril was reluctant to consider it; she equated adopting with the too-painful admission that she was unable to bear her own children. I didn't think the two were mutually

Saturday, July 11

exclusive and told her, "Why not adopt now, and later, if we're lucky, we'll build onto our family with a natural kid? There's no stigma in adopting, and we may as well get on with it while we're prime candidates." Those were my true feelings then, but what I didn't tell her, what I secretly hoped, was that the adoption wouldn't be necessary, because diverting her attention away from conception would mitigate the psychological pressure and lead to pregnancy. It was an academic wrinkle on the old "go away for the weekend with a couple of bottles of wine and relax" routine. I'd heard it happened all the time: couples who'd had trouble conceiving sought instead to adopt, and bang-zoom, the women became pregnant. Even if I was running a bluff, it was a bluff that would please me either way it fell.

I prevailed upon Karril to attend an adoption workshop. It was in our home town, Long Beach; we were one of six couples present. All shared an age range, twenty-seven to thirty-five, the common frustrations of childlessness and the creeping isolation from married couples our age.

On the drive there I got nervous; I wanted to turn around and bag it. But I forced myself to go. The host couple met us at the door and led us downstairs to their basement rec room. We were the last couple to arrive, and when I saw the others my anxiety got the best of me and I lost touch with reality. Objectively, I knew these were normal people confronting the same despondency as Karril and I, but I imagined myself suddenly transported through time and space to that sci-fi bar in the movie *Star Wars,* and I was surrounded by the absolute dregs of the human wine list. To the left of me. The right of me. In front of me. Behind me. A veritable geek-o-rama. Short, bovine geeks. Tall, emaciated geeks. With noses like salamis, teeth like drill bits, and fore-

Saturday, July 11

heads so wide and flat you could land a 747 on them. I had no doubt that this workshop was scheduled at night because none of those people could risk going out in broad daylight for fear of being booked on a 601—offending the public aesthetic.

Where did they round up such a repulsive assembly? Someone must have placed a cast call for a crowd shot in *Swine Flu Fever*. No wonder they're childless. God in His infinite wisdom decided the corruption of the gene pool had gone far enough. This kind of distortion was my method of refusal even to contemplate the possibility that Karril and I were of a piece with all of them, that we fit like a hand in a glove.

It wasn't a workshop in the classical sense of free and open exchange as much as a tutorial on how to engage the cossack horde of the adoption bureaucracy. Although the host couple had adopted successfully, they were extremely cynical about the process. In their view, adoption was the high ground, but the path to it was a mine field. If we got nothing else out of it, we got the message. Their words clung to us like a rash.

Words like: "It's very hard to adopt in this country. You ought to think about going to Mexico or Colombia to get a baby."

Words like: "You have to beware of some agencies. They'll play on your weakness. They'll tell you that there aren't any healthy, normal white infants available now, so first you might want to consider taking an older, handicapped child. It's the bait-and-switch game. The implication is you'll get higher on their waiting list for the next available infant if you're willing to settle for this other child. They do it because they know everyone wants an infant, but their problem is being overstocked with older kids whom nobody wants."

Words like: "We won't give you false hope. The process can take five years, and even then there are no guarantees you'll get what you wanted. Blame it on the pill. Blame it on abortion. Blame it on women keeping their babies. Blame in on whatever makes you feel good. Just remember it's a tight market."

And, perhaps most ironic, considering our immediate circumstance, words like: "A couple sometimes gets so frustrated that they become willing to do anything to get a baby. That's where the Black Market comes in. You can buy a baby if you have enough money. It's illegal, but thousands of couples do it each year. And for some of you it may be the best way to go."

We didn't have our wheels blown off, but by the end of the evening we were certainly wobbling. Without formally scrubbing the idea of adopting we did a *de facto* table job. We didn't call a single adoption agency for the next two years. It looked so hopeless, why bother? So Karril continued to count the days until her supposed ovulation and then go for the gusto, and I continued to bang my head against the wall each time she got her period.

Then, after moving to Washington in hopes of changing our luck for the better, I again pushed adoption, reasoning that a clean start on all fronts included a clean start at getting a baby. By now it was depressingly clear to me that Karril couldn't conceive, and I'd gotten so sick and tired of hearing her whine about being unfulfilled that I told her—in slightly more explicit language than this—to fish, or cut bait. I was blunt: "You want a kid? Then, damn it, go out and get one."

And she tried.

She tried like crazy.

She called adoption services throughout the metropolitan area. Public agencies in D.C.; Alexandria, Virginia; and suburban Montgomery and Fairfax counties.

Saturday, July 11

Private nonsectarian agencies like the Barker Foundation and Peirce-Warwick Adoption Service. Private sectarian agencies representing the Catholic, Lutheran, Episcopalian, and Jewish faiths. Even though none of them offered anything more hopeful than a toehold on the bottom rung of a long ladder, they were all at least cordial. Except one of the local Jewish agencies, which was nasty. After that conversation, Karril came to me with tears in her eyes, saying, "Why would they be so insensitive? Other places don't have babies either, but they didn't make me feel like such a loser." That really hurt, especially considering we were Jewish, and allegedly they were in business specifically to aid people like us. Still, Karril pressed on, making formal application to those agencies that opened their doors just wide enough to allow a letter in.

But my priority remained fixed. No doctor ever told me I was sterile. As far as I knew, I could have my own children. Karril and I often got down to this—that I could, and she couldn't. She regularly offered to leave me, so that I could meet someone else, marry, and have my babies with her. She'd say, "I find it hard to believe you'd rather have me than children. I'm dragging you down with me. You shouldn't have to suffer. I don't want to be selfish."

Not only was her martyrdom disingenuous, but all she was really doing was stretching her passivity to the max by laying the go, no-go call on me. First, she didn't want to go. Second, she'd have been crushed if I'd said, fine, see you around. Third, life isn't a country-western song. So I always told her she was being ridiculous; eventually something would work out for us. But I sometimes hoped she'd hit the road on her own.

I desperately wanted my own child. If not with Karril, then without her. I had this quasi-religious obsession

Saturday, July 11

about blood. If it's in the veins, it counts. If not, you can't ever count on it. My obsession was the legacy of being an only child, of knowing that one day I'd be orphaned. Occasionally I had talked about it with Karril, but I never made her truly understand how consuming the fear was, how it overwhelmed everything I was and hoped to become. With my mother dead and my father past seventy it was out there lying in wait for me. Push came to shove, I felt I couldn't even count on Karril to be there for me. The only way I felt I could ever be connected was to have my own natural child, my own true blood. That's why I couldn't yet commit totally to any adoption. But rather than tell Karril the whole truth and own up to my insecurity, I committed myself partially. If the act was less than honest, at least the intent was noble. To justify it I told myself that Sidney Carton had nothing on me.

She wrote her notes on both sides of a pink sheet of paper: car seat...baby nurse...baby book...wash everything first...kimonos to sleep in...bassinet or port-o-crib...lap pads...diapers—Luvs...Gerber bottle warmer...Playtex bottles...baby brush...will hospital give enough formula for ride home...what kind of formula did baby have in hospital...cloth diapers... receiving blankets, four pkgs...cotton balls...baby lotion...hooded towels...baby washcloths...baby wipes...sterilizing kit.

I looked at them and grinned.

We'd have to get so many things for the trip up to get this kid we might need a U-Haul.

Ted Beitchman had come down from New York to spend the weekend with us, and while Karril was at work he and I spoke about the adoption. I showed him the list. "Look at all this stuff," I said. "There must be $100

Saturday, July 11

worth of junk here, and this is just for the ride home. Well, you know what they say: don't think of it as gaining a child, think of it as taking out a second mortgage."

He didn't laugh. He was pretty good at seeing through my poses under normal circumstances, and now he felt my costume was straight out of the Emperor's New Clothes Fall Catalogue.

"Can you be serious for a while?" he asked.

"Do I have to?"

"Yes."

He asked a lot of good questions, as editors are wont to do. Did I really want this baby? Was I going along with it to please Karril? To help the marriage? When and if the time came to call it off, would the effect on Karril be psychologically and/or physically ruinous? If we did take the baby, could I get beyond the acrid taste of buying it?

I doubted my answers were convincing. On the other hand, what made him Sigmund Freud? I sought his help as a friend, not a marriage counselor.

The three of us went to dinner at Harriet Fier's apartment. Ted and Harriet had worked together at *Rolling Stone* magazine seven years before in San Francisco, and this was a reunion for them. I'd never met Harriet until she came to the *Post* a few months earlier as an editor in the "Style" section, but from our first conversation I sensed an invisible bond gripping us, tying us inextricably together. Although she was from Brooklyn, and I from Long Island, it was as if we'd grown up side by side. Harriet said it didn't matter where I spent my childhood, I "was from the neighborhood." When we talked we were so tuned to the same wavelength that often I felt even closer to her than if she'd been my sister; in fact, I felt that if I'd been born a girl, I'd *be* her. We had

Saturday, July 11

so much in common. Tastes in food, music, movies, writing. Common friends. Common experiences. But the killer was, we even had Karril in common. I didn't think it unusual that Harriet and Karril were born just three days apart. That was a coincidence. But the fact that in 1958—for four weeks and four weeks only—they had been in the same group at day camp, and twenty-three years later, at the instant they met, Karril recognized her and identified their single layer of connective tissue—that was a divine sign. I briefly toyed with not telling Harriet about the adoption, figuring she already knew.

We were all agreed that the adoption was probably illegal, but as long as Karril and I didn't succumb to the seduction of holding the baby in our arms we could continue playing out the scene as we pursued legal protection against the knock on the door. I was gratified that Karril took an active role in the discussion, and particularly intrigued by her thoughts on Polly Westin since she'd never shared them with me before.

I saw the woman as evil. Half-viper, half-vulture. Plots the kill, then picks the carcass. But Karril had no such metaphysical quarrel with Polly; Karril just didn't like her style. "She's trying to pull me, and I don't like being pulled," Karril said. With Karril it was strictly personal. "Polly treats me like I don't know anything and I'm incapable of learning anything except from her. She insists on taking me to a baby store to shop like I'd have no idea what to buy on my own. Well, my sister just had a baby, and she can tell me what to get. She can probably send me some of Jonathan's hand-me-downs. And Polly keeps talking about me getting a nurse, as if I'll be inadequate. I tell her I can get help from my mother, and she tells me that my mother's ideas are outdated. I resent that. What makes her think my mother isn't smart enough or good enough to help, but a total

Saturday, July 11

stranger is? I admit I'm nervous about holding the baby and bathing the baby, but if I have any problems I certainly won't call Polly. I'll call my mother. And anyway, I think the natural instincts will be there with me like with any new mother; I'll know what to do."

I was amazed. Four days into this deal and I'm so juiced I'm popping off all over the lot like a Roman candle, making all sorts of noise and no sort of sense. And here's Karril saying more and saying it more lucidly than I'd ever heard her. So controlled. So sane. So reasonable.

I felt it was too good to be true. I'd known Karril hadn't been sleeping well. Me, I hit the pillow and within ten minutes you can't wake me with a depth charge. But even in good times Karril tosses restlessly, and this week she slept so poorly she woke looking like death warmed over. I'd known she'd been listless at work; she hadn't wanted to wait on customers; when they spoke she often hadn't heard them; she'd wanted to get rid of them quickly so she could sit down; her feet and legs ached. Typically, when she went into one of these cycles she would become moody and withdrawn and ultimately, catatonic. All together these were the external warning signs that she wasn't coping with stress, that it was going straight to her intestines, eating them up inch by inch.

At twenty she'd developed Crohn's disease, an incurable form of colitis which may be, in part, rooted in the psyche. One symptom of Crohn's is chronic diarrhea, a condition that, for obvious reasons, inhibits a full, normal social life. The more the Crohn's separates its victim from the general population, the more psychological strain it provokes, resulting in a downward spiral of systemic destruction that, in Karril's case, possibly exacerbated her difficulty in conceiving. Such was the physical devastation from the disease that at twenty-nine she needed a temporary colostomy. And though the doctors were able to put her back together physically at thirty, no one knew how to patch the hole emotionally. Whatever my reluctance in going through with the adoption, I felt I had to play along for Karril's emotional health. And the signs weren't good. Even with the savvy monologue at dinner, the signs weren't good. I was waiting for the other shoe to drop. And I didn't think it would take long.

After dinner the four of us went to F. Scott's, one of the toniest clubs in Washington. Karril's favorite. Plush, velour booths. Cole Porter tunes on the sound system. Big blown-up posters of movie stars from the forties and fifties on the walls. Elegant black and white motif, tuxedo colors. We were there for more than three hours, and in that span Karril didn't say word one.

The other shoe.

She had gone catatonic.

Sunday, July 12

The good news was that we both had the day off.
The bad news was that we spent it together.
Monday through Saturday our jobs built in routes of escape from the rigors of the baby chase, alleys of digression to wander; there wasn't enough time, as Alexander Haig might say, for an extended confrontative interface. On Sunday there was nothing but time. Even if it was the prudent course under the circumstances, we could hardly choose to spend our lone day together, apart; the implication of such a choice—that we were no longer lovers, only roommates—was too pernicious. So here we were, caged together, and no, the lion didn't lie down with the lamb. He roamed the house like a hungry predator with nothing else to sink his teeth into but his mate. Why is it you always hurt the one you love?
The adoption was a fresh, gaping wound. Letting it fester was suicide; dressing it, homicide. Everything else in our lives was unimportant by comparison, but each time we confronted it, we wound up confronting each other. I couldn't find the right words to make her agree with my position, and she wouldn't use any words at all.
I swore to Karril that I wanted a baby, but this baby was destroying us. I was so persistent, I wound up bullying her. In turn she acted the matador, using her cat-

atonia as a cape to enrage me. Over the course of the day my charges chased her from room to room, and her silence dragged me after her, bouncing off the walls. If I couldn't break through to her, at least I could break something. And then, finally, under the weight of the craziness, I broke. I snapped. The fear and frustration overwhelmed me. I was a thunderclap spending my power in furious shudders, lashing out without thinking. "I've had it, Karril. We're done. I love you, but I can't take another day of this torture. We're killing each other piece by piece over this kid. You've got to pack up, Kar, and get out of here. God, we're dying."

I stormed through her closet, tossing a suitcase out at her, ripping her skirts and blouses from their hangers and flinging them around the bedroom so it looked like the aftermath of a cyclone. "Go to Florida. Go home to your family. You're always telling me how much you miss them anyway, so go to them. Your mother will cater to you like she always does; she'll do everything for you but chew your food. You'll get the goddess treatment. Why have a baby when you can be one? You'll never have to get up in the morning. Never have to work. Never have to hear me scream. Jesus, you'll never even have to speak. Go for it. Don't worry about me. Me and the dog'll do fine."

Through it all Karril sat silent, lifelessly planted at the foot of our bed, head bowed, shoulders sagged, hands clasped in her lap, legs pressed together. Nothing moved but her tears as they followed down, one after the other, the mascara track from her eyes to her cheeks and dropped through the air onto the floor. She was a watercolor dissolving before me.

I may be deliberately cold, but I am not frozen. I started to shiver and sweat simultaneously. There was pain in the center of my chest and my shoulder sockets.

Sunday, July 12

Two hands weren't enough to rub all the sore spots. I thought the top half of my body was going to explode. All I knew for sure was that I didn't want to lose her. Not now. Not this way.

"I'm sorry," I said. "Really, I'm sorry."

I knelt in front of her and touched her hand. She pulled away, refusing to look at me.

"I didn't mean that stuff. Honest, I didn't mean it."

What I saw in her frightened me so, I could hardly speak. And when I did, it came out a mess: "I was, you know, I mean, look, this whole thing has been hard on me, hard on us. We're both under terrific stress. That's some word, 'terrific.' I mean, it's hardly terrific, right?"

She still wouldn't look at me.

"It's just that this thing has gotten me crazy, and I don't know where to take it, you know? Not that I should take it out on you. That's lousy. I'm sorry for that. I'm apologizing. I don't want you to leave. I love you. Honest."

She *still* wouldn't look at me.

I stood up and started pacing the wood floor of the bedroom, trying to get a steady rhythm going to calm the pounding inside my chest. I owed her an explanation. You can't be throwing someone out one second then be begging them to stay the next and pin it all on stress. It just doesn't cut it. I started to wing it.

"The way I look at it," I said, "is that we're together on adoption now, and we weren't before. I mean for years I couldn't be sure you wanted to adopt. Let's face it, Karril, for years you didn't move off the dime. And now it's obvious to me that you're sincere about adopting. I mean you proved it with those calls and letters this past year. But this Polly-Want-A-Cracker Deal, this happened by chance, and I feel like we ought to distinguish between chance and fate. Look, I had nothing to

Sunday, July 12

do with this one, so it's not like we worked together on it, and I think we'd be better off—as a unit I mean—to take a pass on this one and move together on the next one. We'll work through one of the agencies around here, do it nice and kosher. My point is that I feel confident we can really plan the next one out and be totally comfortable with it."

Finally she looked at me.

There were knives in her eyes.

"The *next* one? What are you talking about, the next one?" she asked. She backed me up with her voice. She was hissing. "We wait nine years to have a baby, and now you want to 'take a pass' and wait for the next one? Tony, I don't think you have any idea how tough it was for me to call those adoption agencies."

"I'm sure it was very tough."

"You don't know. You're verbal; words come easily to you. And you can have your own children, so the pain isn't the same." She was still crying, but the provocation had shifted. I wasn't causing these tears. They were coming from a place so deep inside her, I couldn't reach it with an extension cord. "All my life, all I ever wanted was to be a mother. It took me four years to accept that I might not have my own child and make that phone call. Four years to make a call that lasts half a minute, to call up strangers and ask for their help. Ask them for a child, because I was inadequate."

I tried to be encouraging. "Nobody said you were inadequate. It happens to millions of people."

"Shut up, Tony. I'm not talking about millions of people, I'm talking about me. I had to go to them like I was on a job interview. Would they like me enough to let me into their firm? And what do they say? 'Call back in two years, maybe we'll have something then.' They tell you to call the other agencies, and the other agencies

Sunday, July 12

tell you to call other agencies. And then you're supposed to keep calling back once a month for the rest of your life until you get a baby. You know how hard that is for me? Being persistent, calling people like that?"

"Very hard." I felt myself shrinking.

"Once a month? To keep pouring my heart out to strangers? To keep saying it out loud, 'Hi, I can't have my own child. Can you give me one?' It's too hard."

"That's the way it's done, Karril. Nobody ever said it would be easy. We figured on being rejected by most of the agencies."

"But they don't even tell you why. You get a letter in the mail and your fingers are trembling when you go to open it. It's like when you applied to college. It's your number one choice and you haven't been accepted. You call up to ask why, and they won't tell you."

I wanted to be emphathetic. "It's hard on me too. I'm being rejected too."

"Then why do you want to pass on this baby, Tony? Is it the money? I've thought about that. I know it's really a lot of money."

"I worked hard for that money."

"I know. I know it's your money. I know you worked hard for it, and I didn't. How many times are you going to throw that up to me? You think you're buying me this baby as a gift, don't you?"

"Take it easy, Karril. It's not that."

"Because if you think you're buying me the baby then we can't do it. It won't work. It's not a gift, Tony, it's a human life. If you think of it as a gift, you'll never love it. You'll keep looking at the baby as something you bought me, and all you'll see is $15,000."

"I said it's not the money." It really wasn't.

"Then what's this all about?"

I didn't say anything.

Sunday, July 12

Karril asked again, and this time she was demanding an answer. "What's this all about?"

I still didn't say anything. I stood there with my head down, like a bad dog.

I could feel the thought kick into Karril's head with the suddenness of a flare being set off.

"It's one of your tests, isn't it?"

"What do you mean?" I scanned Karril's face. It was the sheer side of a cliff. Nothing there I could grab onto.

"Ever since we've been known each other you've been testing me to see if I really loved you. It was never enough to say it, I always had to pass a test. Because you didn't believe in engagement rings I had to accept not getting one, even though I'd dreamed about one since I was a little girl. All those years when you told me that if I was serious about adopting, I'd do something about it—that was a test too. Because now that I did what you asked, suddenly this baby's not the one you want. Now you want us to forget his one and work together on the next one. Well, did I pass?"

She was wrong. It wasn't a test.

But I didn't know how to tell her that what this was really about was fear. I was *afraid* of this baby, afraid of what it was doing to us.

I wouldn't say the word. So I said nothing.

"I don't know what I should do now," she said. "What do you want me to do? Do you want me to leave you?"

The words hung there. Dead branches.

I moved to her.

"No. Don't leave, Karril. You don't want to go, and I don't want you to. I don't want you to think this was a test, because it wasn't. Try to understand that I have never in my life felt as helpless as this adoption is making me feel. It's making me nuts, Karril. Please, let's forget about what just happened. Forget that I tried to throw

Sunday, July 12

you out. Forget that you offered to go. Forget my accusations. Forget yours. Let's just try as best we can to get through this thing together. Let's not throw nine years of marriage down the drain. I'll try my best to smooth things out from now on. Will you try too? Will you try with me?"

Thirteen years ago this week we had our first date, and since then there had never been another girl for me or another boy for her. Was it fear of being alone which held us together? Was it habit? There were rips in our marriage as in everyone's. But if marriage is a quilt woven over time, surely love is the stitching.

She took my hand and held on.

Monday, July 13

Back at work, I started my research for a profile of Representative John LeBoutillier (R-N.Y.), at twenty-eight years old the youngest member of Congress. Unlike most of his colleagues who can go twenty years in office without so much as casting a shadow, LeBoutillier had taken just six months to become notorious as the Mouth of the House. Plunging to an enviable depth in the ooze of partisan politics, LeBoutillier charged that the Speaker of the House, Tip O'Neill, was "big, fat, and out of control." On the bipartisan front LeBoutillier concluded that his fellow Republican, the chairman of the Senate Foreign Relations Committee, Charles Percy, was "a wimp." I wanted to write about Le Boutillier because he was a trailblazer; America's first punk congressman.

Step one on a profile is to check the clips. You go to your newspaper's library, or "morgue," where the paper has collected and filed every story ever printed on its pages about the subject. Newspapers of record, like the *Washington Post* and the *New York Times,* flesh out their inventory with material from other papers and magazines; the clip file on someone like Richard Nixon is thicker than gravy at a college cafeteria. There wasn't a lot on LeBoutillier; he'd only been a newsworthy figure for a brief time. Since I had nothing pressing, and rather than begin the hard reporting on him—checking his

Monday, July 13

financial disclosures, calling political sources—I chose to do some personal reading, and I pulled the *Post's* clips on adoption. Stacks of them. They took the entire morning to sift through.

It didn't surprise me to find many references to Black Market adoptions. As far back as 1963 Senator Estes Kefauver introduced legislation to outlaw them. It obviously hadn't passed since there are not now, nor have there ever been, federal statutes governing adoption. What was particularly intriguing about the Kefauver story, though, was the identification of twelve states—including those currently relevant to my situation, New York, New Jersey, and Maryland—and the District of Columbia as areas which Kefauver said had "serious problems" with Black Market adoption trafficking. The rate ceilings, according to Kefauver, were "in Arizona as high as $1,000 and in California as high as $7,000." One year later, witnesses testifying before the Senate Subcommittee on Juvenile Delinquency estimated that a Black Market adoption cost as much as $7,500.

By 1976, three years after the Supreme Court decision legalizing abortion, America was on the cutting edge of oil embargoes and double-digit inflation, and testimony before the Senate Subcommittee on Children and Youth placed the top price of a Black Market adoption at $20,000 and the annual number of children thus adopted at 4,000. The next year, in a hearing before a Congressional panel looking into such illegal practices, Joseph V. Morello, an assistant district attorney in Manhattan, put the price for a healthy, white infant as high as $25,000. And in 1981, Bill Pierce of the National Committee for Adoption said that in California, the fast lane of the country, Black Market babies were being sold for as much as $40,000. Healthy, white infants were almost as expensive as Malibu beach houses.

Monday, July 13

Many of the clips were short, wire service items. Adoption oddities. Your basic Freak of the Week story: Long Island judge refused to allow sixty-year-old man and fifty-five-year-old wife to adopt their four-year-old foster child because judge sought a "more contemporary environment" for child; Kingston, New York couple of Italian extraction successfully sue to adopt blond child after being denied permission by adoption agency on grounds they were too darkly complected to suitably raise child; Iowa woman denied custody of her natural twin daughters because her IQ said to be too low; New Jersey couple refused permission to adopt because they admit not believing in God; Pittsburgh adopted siblings ordered not to marry although not biologically related; Detroit judge rejected petition of a childless couple to pay surrogate to give birth to baby they plan to adopt; D.C. woman, during her trial but prior to conviction for killing one and beating her two other adopted children, given yet a fourth child to adopt.

Then there was the Guaranteed to Bring Tears of Joy (or Pain) human interest group. In this category was the Natural Parent (or Child) Seeks Reunion with Dislocated Child (or Parent) story. One such plea, written by a natural mother, using a pseudonym of course, bleats, "We do have needs. We are human. This is to you, my son, whatever your name is and wherever you are. I still love you, and I would like to hold you, just once."

These stories really make me puke. They invariably disregard the emotional price paid by the adoptive parents—the only real parents the child has known—when some bimbo waltzes in after God only knows how many years and says, "Hi baby, Mommy's home." Where was she when little Timmy lost his first tooth? Or when he fell off his bike and needed stitches? Or when his dog

Monday, July 13

died? The bleeding-heart feature writers of the world beat their breasts and howl that natural parents have been cheated out of such a *profound* relationship. Bull. You don't show up for practice, you don't play in the game. And these stories discount the trauma facing adoptive parents on the inevitable day their child, his emotional system overloaded with angst, drops the bomb: "You aren't my real parents. I'm leaving to find my roots. I've got to know who I really am." Actually, he has it backwards. The people he's searching for were only his genetic surrogates; the people he's abandoning are his true family. It's a false promise, the achieving of inner peace simply by nursing on the biological root.

It's disheartening that so many crimes of journalistic excess are committed in the name of human interest. Not that everything in the clips came from either the freak file or the puff patch. There were some hard news reporting on the Baby Lenore DeMartino custody case and on Bobby Burns's Florida baby farm. But in the main the feature stories reflected larger cultural patterns. The clips from 1965 to 1974, encompassing Lyndon Johnson's Great Society initiative and the socio-political consciousness of the Woodstock generation, were dominated by stories about interracial and special-needs adoptions; from 1975 to 1977, in the guilt-ridden aftermath of the Vietnam War, and with Southeast-Asian boat people drilling holes in our national psyche, the files overflowed with stories about wholesale *noblesse oblige* adoptions of Vietnamese and Cambodian children; from 1978 to 1981, as the fight to ratify the Equal Rights Amendment and a baby boom among couples over thirty focused attention on traditional concepts of sexual and family roles, the files were stuffed with stories about searches for natural parents and adopted children

Monday, July 13

and the conflict between the principle of absolute secrecy in adoption proceedings and the civil rights of the individuals involved.

Of the hundreds of clips I ran through, there were two that ran through me: one was a 1977 story out of Pennsylvania describing a Black Market adoption ring devised and operated by lawyers. These legal eagles stocked their shelves by setting up a phony abortion counselling clinic. They paid hospital nurses and lab technicians to direct young, unmarried women who appeared distressed about being pregnant to this particular clinic. There the "counsellors" offered up to $10,000 to those women they thought would be receptive to continuing their pregnancies, then signing over their babies to the lawyers who would place them for adoption. The lawyers then sold the babies for up to $30,000. A rather neat turnkey operation until the police moved in.

The other was a 1981 story out of Texas concerning an adoption agency that had exhausted its waiting list and announced it would accept applicants for the twenty to thirty babies it anticipated placing in the next year. Applicants were told to come in person on a Thursday morning. By Wednesday evening 200 couples, some from as far away as Arkansas and Oklahoma, had lined up outside the agency, perfectly content to sleep out in the cold for a chance to adopt a baby.

In the afternoon I hit the phones again. I reached Peter Sherman, a Washington lawyer whose name I'd gotten from the *Post*'s legal counsel, Bo Jones. I gave Sherman no indication that my inquiry into how to legally adopt a child in the District was anything other than a reporter seeking background information for a story. He said the adopter needs explicit consent from both parties, father and mother. Since Grace had already told me that the

Monday, July 13

father was agreeable to the adoption I didn't think that would be a problem. "And there can't be any brokering involved. It can't be in the nature of selling a baby," Sherman said. "No doctors and no lawyers can be involved in arranging the adoption. Any adoption that smacked of that wouldn't be proper in the District. The issue is remuneration."

If that information brought me near the edge, what I got next sent me right to it. Deborah Luxenberg called and addressed the technical interpretation of brokering, citing the 1976 *District of Columbia* v. *Galison* case.

Edward Galison was a Long Island lawyer who came to D.C. to pick up an infant boy from his natural mother who had herself come to D.C. from Florida with her mother to give birth. According to published reports Galison had previously agreed to pay the natural mother's medical expenses and the two women's living expenses while in D.C., an amount that Galison said totalled $4,000, in return for the baby, whom he planned to deliver to an adoptive couple waiting in New York.

But after the birth the natural mother didn't want to give up her son, and she contacted D.C. authorities and explained the deal she had made, asserting that Galison was not only paying $2,000 in legitimate expenses but also giving her a $2,000 cash bonus. A sting operation was set up and the natural mother was told to go along with the original arrangement. After Galison took the baby from George Washington University Hospital he was arrested by D.C. police and charged not with buying a baby, but with violating the Baby Brokers Act, which provides the legal method for adopting in D.C. It reads, in part, "No person other than the parent, guardian, or relative within the third degree, and no firm, corporation, association, or agency, other than a licensed child-placing agency, may place or arrange or assist in placing or arranging for the placement of a child under sixteen years of age in a family home or for adoption."

Galison's lawyer argued that Galison was licensed to arrange adoptions in New York, that he was ignorant of any breach of D.C. law and meant no harm by his actions. But Galison was convicted of the misdemeanor offense, fined $300 and given a suspended sentence.

The law didn't allow room to maneuver. "In a direct adoption, such as the one you're describing," Luxenberg told me, "the only parties that can be involved are the people who want to adopt the child and either the natural mother or an immediate relative or guardian of the natural mother. Under the Baby Brokers Act you have to deal with them directly. Whoever else you go through is violating the law."

I felt certain that Polly Westin and Grace Zimmer were culpable, and I asked, "Would the foster mother qualify as a guardian?"

"Not if it was the informal relationship you described."

That meant Judy Amalfitano was culpable too.

"And the penalties?"

"The seller, not the buyer, is criminal."

That was wonderful news. I should have hung up then and there, because the rest of what Luxenberg said wasn't so wonderful: "Once you petition for adoption, the District will investigate the circumstances of the adoption before granting a final decree, and they will contact the mother or a relative to determine if the law was upheld. The problem is, is it a valid adoption? D.C. is very uptight about direct placements. They don't want them, except through agencies. Whenever they can stop direct adoptions, they will."

She said she was sorry to be so discouraging.

Monday, July 13

I told her to forget it. Forewarned is forearmed.

I was ready to tell Karril all about it. I was sure there was no way we could follow their plan and have a valid adoption; I couldn't let Karril cling to an unreasonable hope.

But since we'd gone this far, why not go a little farther? Why not try and pressure them to modify the arrangements? I figured we already had enough on Polly, Grace, and Amalfitano to at least get them arrested, which would be terribly embarrassing for them. There was no shot they were going to push us around anymore.

I was really pumped up. I sat at my desk and considered how to maximize the theatrical effect when I reached the part about having these creeps by the short hairs. I decided on the King Kong pose; I'd extend my right arm, my hand palm up as if holding dried leaves, and tell Karril that any time I chose to, I could crush them.

After work I went across the street from the *Post* to the back bar at the Madison Hotel for a couple of birthday drinks with some friends from the "Style" section. While I was there, Polly Westin came to visit the house, bringing her four-year-old adopted daughter. Karril showed them around and did some general entertaining for forty-five minutes, then joined me downtown for the tail end of the happy hour. It wasn't until we got home that we talked about Polly's visit. Why spoil a party?

"She was disappointed you weren't here," Karril said.

"She can go straight to Hell," I said. I hated Polly. I thought she was the lowest, most corrupt kind of user there was, the kind who makes a profit off someone's unhappiness and vulnerability. A parasite. A blight. "She brought her adopted kid, huh?" I pantomimed a fisherman hauling in a big one. "The woman has no shame."

"I guess she wanted to see how I'd react. To see if I could handle it."

"I thought we were going to try to do it at her house?"

"You knew she wouldn't agree to that. She came here to check us out."

"So, did we pass inspection?"

"I think so. The house was clean. She seemed to like it."

"Give her the grand tour?"

"Yeah. I took her through the house, showed her the rooms. She wanted to see where we'd put the baby, and I brought her up to the guest room. It was really hot and humid, but she saw the air conditioner and told me to use it when we got the baby so the baby would be comfortable. I took her into the backyard and told her I could bring the baby out to sit in the fresh air. But she thought it was too buggy for a baby."

I did my best Jimmy Durante. "Everybody's a critic."

"She liked the porch better. She said that would be good for the baby."

"Then what?"

"Then we went into the living room and chatted. She kept telling me that we had to go out to Crib N' Cradle to look at baby things. She's got this thing about us shopping together. Every time I talk to her she mentions it."

"Maybe she's got stock in the company."

"Well, it upsets me."

"Why?"

"Because we really don't have anything for a baby."

"So we'll get stuff. How tough is it to whip out a Visa card and buy a crib?"

"That's not what I mean. The guest room's much too big for a baby. Maybe if I had time I could do something

Monday, July 13

with it. But what am I going to have? A week? Ten days? I'm good at knitting. I could have knitted a blanket, or made a mobile like I did for Jonathan. A pregnant woman gets nine months to prepare."

I smiled. "We'll make it up to the kid later on. If you start now, you can knit him a car for his seventeenth birthday."

She giggled.

"Anything else happen?" I asked.

"Not much. Oh, she said she wants me to come to her house and see her four-month-old, her natural daughter. She wants to show me how to bathe her. She started talking about how she puts cotton in her navel before putting her in the water. It was crazy. I think if I stick around her long enough I'll become a terribly neurotic mother."

"She's a couple of quarts low, huh?"

"I don't know. She seemed friendly enough. Kind of warm. I expected her to be pushy, and she wasn't. When I showed her the rooms I thought she'd walk through and just take over. She didn't. But I still didn't trust her. The only reason she was here was business. After we get this baby I don't want any part of her."

"Fine with me. I don't want any part of her now." I started into the kitchen to look for something to nibble on. "By the way, she say anything that seemed odd? Anything we ought to be concerned about?"

Karril's face looked like she'd been sniffing drainpipes. "Actually, yes. It was weird. She was getting ready to go and she said, 'Now that I've met you I can say that you're my friend. But I can't say that yet about your husband.'"

"What the hell does that mean? The woman has to certify me? What is she, a notary public?"

"I think it's just another one of her games. If I'm her

friend then what she's doing isn't really selling me a baby; friends don't sell babies to friends. I think it's a technicality that allows her to lie to herself about the whole thing."

We were lying in bed when it occurred to me that I had no idea what any of them looked like. Three women out there were pulling the strings of my life like I was some kind of puppet, and I hadn't even put faces on them.

I thought about my own looks: 6 feet tall, 185 pounds. Certainly not fat, but maybe a bit flabby around the middle. Blue eyes. Brown hair. Though not much of it. The genetic chips were cashed and I was balding. Blondish mustache. Pale skin. Large red nose. People saw me and assumed I was a big drinker because my face always resembled a ripe tomato. Not an ugly face, but by no means a handsome one.

And I thought about Karril's looks: small, fragile, 5-2, 95. Tie a long ribbon to her waist and in a strong wind you've got a kite. Because of the cortisone drugs she had to take her face was puffy, but her skin was soft and smooth. Thick brown hair. Large brown eyes. And still so very cute and youthful. Like a chipmunk.

Then I tried to put a face on Polly. But nothing popped into my mind.

So I tried to put a face on Grace. Again, nothing popped.

Only Amalfitano came fully assembled. I imagined her dusky, with eyebrows thick enough to use as oven mitts, and the trace of a mustache by the corners of her mouth. Pear-shaped, but soft only from the neck down; her face would be severe, like distressed oak. I saw her as an extra in an Anthony Quinn war movie, reclining in a black bean-bag chair, the lumpy folds of her black

Monday, July 13

caftan melting into the lumpy folds of the chair's vinyl covering. She was absolutely still. The only piece of her that moved was her eyes, which darted around, not missing a thing. She was a boa constrictor, and she frightened me.

I nudged Karril. "I forgot to ask you what Polly looked like," I said. "Tell me what she looked like."

"She was tall," Karril said, half asleep.

"How tall?"

"Five-eight, maybe 5–9."

I waited for more. It wasn't forthcoming.

"That's all?" I asked. "Just tall? Nothing else?"

"I don't know," Karril said, keeping her eyes closed. "She was in her mid-thirties, maybe thirty-three, thirty-four. She had a nice figure. She was wearing a sundress, and she had frosted hair that she did in a tight perm. She was perky. She looked like your typical suburban Jewish housewife. Okay?"

"Nothing distinctive?"

"Yeah. Her eyelashes."

"Her eyelashes? What about them?"

"They were false. She wore false eyelashes. Nobody wears false eyelashes anymore. They've been out for ten years."

Karril rolled over and went back to sleep.

I looked at the clock on my night table. It was close to 1 A.M. It was already tomorrow; my birthday was history. It had come and gone without a phone call from Grace.

The baby hadn't been born on my birthday.

I took it as a divine sign.

Tuesday, July 14

What do Moses, Gerald Ford, and Son of Sam have in common?

You get three guesses.

They were Bernardo in their high-school productions of *West Side Story*?

No.

They shave with an electric razor?

No.

They play the trombone?

No. They were adopted.

It's true.

Just as it's true that adopted children display a general increase in their levels of intellectual functioning as well as in physical health following the adoption.

Just as it's true that the ancient Chinese held that a childless married male was entitled to claim and adopt the firstborn male child of his younger brother.

Just as it's true that adoption is the societal norm in the Polynesian Marquesa Islands, where a pregnant woman receives requests from other islanders who desire to raise her child, and within a few months of the birth she places the infant with one of the petitioners.

I found all this information and more in the books and magazine articles I pulled from the stacks at the Library of Congress this morning before going to work.

Tuesday, July 14

Over three hours I read all or parts of *Let's Talk about Adoption* by Susan and Elton Klibanoff; "The Infertile Couple" by Barbara Menning; *A Parent's Guide to Adoption* by Robert S. Lasnik; "Where Have All the Children Gone?" by Marie Hoeppner; "Children: A Factor in Marital Satisfaction" by Eleanore Luckey and Joyce Baim; "Study of Adopted Children" by Anna Elonen and Edward Schwartz, and *Beyond the Best Interests of the Child* by Joseph Goldstein.

I like going to the Library of Congress anytime, but especially on hot summer days when it is literally one of the coolest places in Washington to visit. Owing to its marble-and-tile construction, it can be 98 degrees with 95 percent humidty outside—stickier than cheating on your wife with her best girlfriend—but down in the stacks you'll need a sweater. I liked the irony of being there today, researching what for me posed a potential judicial problem. Because next door to the Library of Congress on First Street N.E. is the Supreme Court building, and I'd like to think that someday soon those three Macbethian witches—Polly Westin, Grace Zimmer, and Judy Amalfitano—will be there, losing their final appeal before being carted off to the slammer for selling babies.

I walked to my car having taken ten pages of delicate notes with a blue felt-tip pen on a yellow legal pad. And on page two of those ten there was a quote from "The Infertile Couple" which I had transcribed in fine, flowing script and underlined in red ink: "Armed with false hopes, the infertile couple may rush into a frantic search for an adopted baby. They may be pathetically confused, and desperate."

I wondered how that would look in needlepoint.

Back at the office I worked the phone. Since Dan Lauck was working on pinning down an address and phone number for Amalfitano through his FBI contact, I concentrated on Polly and Grace. I wanted to see if they were playing straight with me, so I matched the telephone numbers they'd given me with the numbers and addresses in the directory. I wan't exactly sure what a discrepancy would prove, but I was sure that it would bother me to find one. Polly checked out fine. The number she had given us corresponded to the one listed under her husband's name. Grace didn't check out so fine. The number she had given us didn't match either of the listed numbers at her address, under her name or her husband's, or their initials. And the operator said there were no unpublished numbers at that address. It seemed likely she had given us a business number to call. But whose name was it registered under? I wondered if it might be a Gray Market network number funded by baby sales. It was a real long shot, but if indeed there was any such association with that number the long-distance logs could be dynamite in any judicial proceeding.

While I drooled over that possibility I got a return call from Sherry Bindeman, Sidney Sachs's associate. Sachs had only limited knowledge of adoption law so he was recommending I contact a Washington lawyer named Leslie Scherr. Scherr was not only the ranking expert in town on adoption law, but he had adopted children of his own. I immediately called his office to set up an appointment, but his secretary said he was tied up for the rest of the day and he would get in touch with me tomorrow.

I was hopeful that Scherr would be my ticket in Washington, but I wanted to keep all my options open so I called a friend in New York, a lawyer named Jerry Davis, one of those rare and gifted people who could deliver so many quality services that he ought to have multiple

Tuesday, July 14

listings in the Yellow Pages. I told him I needed someone up there who knew adoption law inside and out in case I tried to do the adoption in New York where I still voted and owned property. He gave me the name of a Rochester lawyer, Donna Finnegan.

I called and briefed her on my situation. Motive. Money. Mystery. When I mentioned the term, Gray Market, she took over.

"Gray Market will take a check; you're dealing with Black Market," she said authoritatively. "What do you know about the child's health? How much information can you get on the mother?"

"Only what we're told," I said.

"And you can't corroborate it, can you?"

I said, "No," but I knew it was asked rhetorically. There was something in Donna Finnegan's approach which told me she had been down this road before; I could almost feel her wince through the wires as she spoke.

"Then, for all intents and purposes it's like a Third-World Child," she said. "You pay your money and take your chances."

Encouraging, it wasn't. "What do I need for protection?"

"The natural mother must sign the consent forms herself. Don't take them if this foster mother signs. Pay no attention to anything she says about having power of attorney. Power of attorney doesn't mean a thing. Get the papers in hand before the transfer."

"And if I can't?"

"Look, I can't tell you what to do on this. In the adoption scene everyone's a potential victim. But you're especially vulnerable without the legal work in order. I'm afraid that once you hand over the cash you're in trouble. Then again, if you make waves, the baby will disappear. Just disappear, and you'll never even get close."

So much for me crushing them.

"Who's getting the money?" I asked.

"Probably everybody involved," she said. "But you already suspected that, didn't you?"

"Well how am I supposed to get a lawyer to represent me in this?"

"You'll have to lie about the money."

I already suspected that too. "So assuming we do it, and assuming we can get away with it, what's the biggest risk we face with the kid?"

"Genetic." I knew from the way she said it, from her quiver, that I wasn't going to feel good about what was coming, that she had a story to tell that was going to sound like bones breaking. I took a deep breath and tried to get ready.

"Six years ago my husband and I went to Colombia to adopt a little girl," she said. "Before we left, some friends who'd been through a similar experience told us that there were two things we absolutely had to remember: we might not get the exact baby we were going down for. But under no circumstances were we to come back without a baby.

"We had been told that our baby was a three-week-old girl, and we'd been asked by one of the women who ran the orphanage there to bring down a small doll. It struck me as odd because it was a very specific request for an expensive imported doll. But I assumed it was for the orphanage, and in addition to the doll I brought down clothes and toys. I ought to explain that the women who ran this orphanage were the aristocrats of Colombia, the wives of government and military leaders,

Tuesday, July 14

very wealthy, cultured women with huge houses and servants. I assumed that this was their charitable endeavor, that they were doing a noble thing by giving these poor Colombian orphans a chance at a better life in America. But when I got there and saw what was really going on, I was shocked. It was hard for me to believe these women weren't running a retail shop. The orphanage was stocked with hand-embroidered dresses from Spain, boxes and boxes of Pampers, leather photograph albums, Fisher-Price toys, imported dolls, and stuffed animals. And none of these things were for the orphans. They were for the children of these aristocratic women. They were payoffs. Sure, when you got there the women offered to reimburse you for the gifts you brought. But no one would dare take any money for fear of offending them.

"In addition, when we arrived we learned through the semiofficial grapevine that we were expected to make a donation, in cash or money order, to the orphanage. But not in Colombian currency. We were even asked if we would cash some checks that other Americans had written to the orphanage. Nobody ever said how much we should give, and we didn't want to give too much for fear of pushing the standard up too high. But we didn't know how much was too much. It was obvious that the money would go straight into their pockets, but what could we do? You're in a foreign country; the rules are different. If you don't play along, you may not get your child.

"I think the most depressing realization was how thoroughly guileful the entire operation was. The orphanage we visited was really just a clearinghouse. The children didn't actually live there. They were collected from the real orphanages and brought there to be transferred. We

Tuesday, July 14

got there on a Friday and were told, 'A shipment is coming in this afternoon. Come back on Monday and we'll have a baby for you.' A 'shipment.' I mean, how crass is that? They never let us near a real orphanage. I can only imagine they were so squalid they would have mortified us."

I felt I had to say something.

"How did you feel about all this?"

"How did we feel? We were in shock."

"This gets worse, doesn't it?"

"Much."

She was speaking rapidly, as if she was facing some sort of deadline. I had the feeling that if she couldn't get it out in one big burst the words would stick in her throat and strangle her. I listened for the tears that I knew were coming.

"The child they gave us had been born premature. She didn't look healthy, but we knew this was the Third World, that babies didn't come eight pounds and up, so we took her back to the hotel where we were staying. We wanted to get more background on her birth, but we knew that if we pressed them for facts they'd just make something up. The next day we took her to a Spanish-speaking doctor the orphanage recommended and brought our cab driver with us to translate. We were nervous because the baby seemed to have something wrong in one eye and she was having diarrhea. The doctor examined her and said she was fine. But a few days later she hadn't improved and we found an English-speaking doctor and brought her there. He told us she was seriously dehydrated and might not live. He immediately placed her in a hospital he was affiliated with. The next morning we learned the baby already had a serious urinary infection and had suffered convulsions. The doctor thought she might have spinal men-

Tuesday, July 14

ingitis. He told us, 'This baby is at very high risk. Do not adopt this baby.'

"We were heartsick. We were afraid that if we took her home with us, she might die on the plane. So we went back to the orphanage and told them what had happened and that we didn't think we should take this baby. They were furious. Apparently we had humiliated them by seeing this English-speaking doctor. It turned out that he was familiar with their shoddy placements, and had made similar recommendations to other American couples. Meanwhile we found out that the doctor the orphanage had originally sent us to wasn't a pediatrician at all, but a retired military surgeon.

"I remembered the warning we had been given before going down to Colombia, that under no circumstances were we to return without a child. So I asked the women for another baby.

"They said, 'We won't have another one for months.'

"Well, we were crushed. We were a childless couple, and just like you we wanted a child more than anything in the world. We didn't know what to do. We went back to our hotel and called the English-speaking doctor. Fortunately he was able to convince the women to give us another baby, and we went back to the orphanage and were given the child who is our present daughter."

If this story was to end happily Donna Finnegan would have stopped here.

She didn't.

"My daughter developed epilepsy at four," she said.

And now the tears I knew would come, were here.

"She lost all her speech. She'll probably never speak again. She is brain damaged now. But we didn't know that then. All we knew then was that she had scabs on her head, which we thought was par for the course down there. We took her to another English-speaking doctor.

Tuesday, July 14

He examined the scabs and said they were just sebaceous cysts. She really seemed to be in better shape than most of the children that are adopted from Colombia. She had no parasites. Most do. The doctor's overall diagnosis was that she was just malnourished, and it was amazing to see how she responded to a proper diet. We could actually see the shape of her face change from food."

"Why did you take her?" I asked softly.

"I don't know. I don't think we were able to assess the risk. I wanted so much to have a child."

"When did the problems begin to show?"

"She was slow learning to speak. Our neurologist in New York says she's had brain damage all along."

"Do you think the Colombian doctor knew?"

"No. He couldn't have known. The etiology was such that you couldn't have predicted it until you saw something manifest itself."

"You must feel terribly cheated." I didn't want to push, but I felt we'd gone down so far we might as well touch bottom.

"We were in such shock for the first year of this that I couldn't get to that." She was more composed now. "Ultimately I felt rage. Rage. Over the years it dissipated into a kind of sadness."

For a few seconds she said nothing, and I waited. When she spoke again her voice was soaked by such a torrent of tears that I thought a dam had burst inside of her.

"We always felt God wanted us to go there and have her. We've never lost that. She belongs here. If we had left her there, she would've died in the streets somewhere, in a grand mal seizure." She was sobbing uncontrollably. "Please excuse me," she finally said. "It's

Tuesday, July 14

just been so long since I've spoken about this. I'm sorry."

"Believe me, I understand. I don't mean to torture you."

"No, it's okay." She was putting herself back together again. "You asked me before if I felt cheated? There are times I do, yes. I continue to do adoption work, and when I see American couples adopt a Colombian child who isn't damaged, somewhere that hits me. But the apparatus down there still has terrible cracks. I know a woman who recently went down there to adopt siblings, but when she got there she was told that the children she had come for weren't available. Out of nowhere they produced a new boy and girl for her. They said the girl was four, but when she had the girl examined by a doctor here she found out the girl was really seven or eight; her development was so stunted she just looked four. And to top it off, they weren't even brother and sister."

"Jesus." I felt punctured.

"Look, I know you're not going to South America to adopt. And I don't tell you all this to discourage you." There was empathy in her voice now. "I know what it's like not to have children. I know the pain. I wish you all the luck in the world. I just want you to go in with your eyes open. Protect yourself. Try and minimize the risks."

I knew I was treading on thin ice, but there was one more thing I wanted to know. "If you don't mind, what happened to the original baby they gave you?"

"We took her to the hospital and arranged to pay all her medical bills while they treated her."

"Did you see her again?"

"No."

"Do you have any idea what happened to her? I mean, is it possible she's not alive now?"

Tuesday, July 14

I could tell from the moan that I had gone too far, unlocked a door I had no business even knocking on.
"Yes, it's quite possible."
I thanked her for her time, her story, and her advice. When I hung up the phone my whole body was shaking.

I called Grace at the work number she'd given me. I didn't ask her to explain why the home number she'd given me didn't correspond to the ones the telephone operators gave out. I never challenged Grace. I was always solicitous of her, even obsequious. Whereas I sensed that Polly was merely a local agent and therefore auxiliary to this adoption, I was convinced that since Grace would physically transfer the baby to me, she was crucial and needed to be handled with the utmost care. I based my entire strategy, such as it was, on the assumption that I was smarter than the people I was forced to deal with, and that in the end my only shot was to out think them.

I told Grace that while I hadn't as yet hired a lawyer, I had received counsel to the effect that the natural father's consent was necessary, and that we should have all the proper consent forms in hand prior to picking up the baby. I wanted her to ask Amalfitano to be present at the transfer, explaining that we would like to meet her and thank her for all she had done; I carefully omitted the real reason I wanted her there—so I could take her picture and keep it as evidence. And while she was talking to Amalfitano, could she try and get the name of the social worker assigned to the natural mother's case? My stated reason was that our lawyer might require the name, but again I kept my real motivation hidden; I thought the social worker might be getting a piece of the action and I wanted the name for any future

Tuesday, July 14

legal inquiry. Even if the social worker was ignorant of the monetary arrangement, such testimony in and of itself might be useful to counteract any claim of coercion filed by the natural mother.

I was asleep when Grace called back at eleven-thirty. Karril spoke with her. Grace said she had done some checking, and because the natural mother was unmarried, the natural father's formal consent was unnecessary. Grace did not have the name of the social worker, but she said our lawyer could get it through W. Allan Cavas. Regarding consent forms, Grace said we would get them when we picked up the baby. Not before. Judy Amalfitano would bring the baby to Grace's house, but she would not be present for the transfer. Case closed.

When Karril finished relaying all this information, I realized we were in a cat and mouse game with a leopard. But my sense of things was irrelevant to Karril, who was preoccupied only with what Grace had told her about the natural mother's condition: she had begun to dilate, and was scheduled to go to her doctor and take a fetal stress test within forty-eight hours. A caesarean section would be performed if necessary, but since her water hadn't broken yet, the birth was still thought to be two or three days away.

Grace's last words to Karril were, "Everything looks fine."

Wednesday, July 15

Children can't save a marriage.

A marriage stands or falls under the weight of the relationship between husband and wife; children are, ultimately, separate issues. If the cracks go too deep, a marriage eventually collapses no matter what steps are taken to shore it up. At best, adopting a child only patches the damage temporarily.

I wanted to be a father. Karril wanted to be a mother.

But not to save our marriage.

Our marriage already had lasted nine years, and given our psychological dynamics, it would likely last another twenty-nine. Infertility had put a significant strain on the marriage, but it hadn't dealt a mortal blow. So the act of adopting a child wasn't to save our marriage. We had obviously proven that we could survive without a child. And we could survive without this child. What scared me was that the *process* by which we wouldn't adopt this child could be so bloody that it would destroy our marriage. If ever we had to think with one mind and speak with one voice it was now.

Admittedly we were not Ozzie and Harriet. But despite our routine bitching we were actually getting along pretty well now. I was Roman candling with less frequency; the more accustomed to the chase I became, the less manic I acted. Karril and I found enough common

Wednesday, July 15

ground to agree that modification of the plan, specifically as regarded the $15,000 cash payment, would have to be effected. We also agreed on a basic overall strategy: we would not antagonize Grace or Polly; we would continue to make them think that we were the right, indeed the *only* choice for this child. That way we would make them dependent on us to follow through. When they finally put the baby in our arms, the last thing they could expect would be our willingness to give it back and walk away empty-handed. So, when the time for decisive action came, we would take them completely by surprise by dictating new terms on the spot, forcing an immediate contest of wills. Call, or fold. If they didn't have a backup family we might steal the pot on a bluff.

But all this maneuvering was not without its psychic cost. I always had doubts about Karril's resolve. In the matter of babies I had come to see her as emotional beachfront; subjected to heavy wind and rain she was likely to erode. I feared that after the child was born—when there was a definite "he" or "she," not this disembodied "it"—Karril's nerves would go into a full-tilt boogie and her commitment to our strategy would dissolve.

On the other hand, I knew I too was posing. Worse, I was lying. To cement our alliance I regularly assured Karril that I wanted this baby, that I was certain we would work something out. But I only gave her my number; I never gave her my situation.

If she pressed me on why I put so much emotional distance between myself and the adoption, I just peeled away the top layer, that I had no respect for the procedure: "Ever since I started working on newspapers I've told myself that the socially redemptive aspect of being a journalist was in catching the crooks. Now, when it's to my personal benefit to do so, I'm doing business with them. I'm a real paragon of virtue and ethics, aren't I? In order to get a lawyer I have to lie about the money and how the adoption was set up. So I'm not only a willing accomplice, entering into an illegal conspiracy with premeditation, but my lack of full disclosure puts my lawyer at risk for perjury and disbarment. After that, how in the hell am I supposed to climb up on a white horse? I mean, where's my credibility? Christ, I'm one of the bad guys. We're buying a baby here. Any way you cut it we're breaking the law."

My position was passionate and convincing. And, it was true, as far as it went. But I knew it didn't speak to the core of the problem, which was that I didn't yet have any real feeling for this kid.

The issue of parenting seemed to be different for Karril and me.

I wanted a child.

I felt she needed one.

I had other things going on. Good friends. A good job that in a given month might take me to places like Los Angeles, Houston, and New York, might put me face-to-face with people like Tip O'Neill, Muhammad Ali, and Paul Newman. Obviously, I'm star-tripping here for effect. I don't mean to suggest that the regular glamour of my work seduced me into defining myself by the places I went or the people I interviewed; I may be shallow, but I'm not flat. But clearly I get enough back that, on balance, I thought my life was basically good. And it was full enough that I could go for months without being overwhelmed by my childlessness. My identity wasn't solely determined by not being a parent.

But without a child Karril seemed to have no identity. It was as if she'd banked her whole sense of self on becoming a mother. In that respect she was far removed from most women her age, college educated

Wednesday, July 15

in the sixties and card-carrying Libbers. Their aspirations weren't her aspirations. Their issues weren't her issues. It had always troubled me that Karril disdained the social and political values of our generation, that my wife seemed so different from my friends' wives. I may well have resisted the application of equality within our marriage, but I damned sure endorsed the principle. Why she never fought for it, why she never even *wanted* it disheartened me. Often I felt we'd grown up in different eras. She was far more a child of the fifties than the sixties. Out of touch. Out of step. Out of time. Her concept of womanhood was tied to staying home and raising children, just like her mother. And like her mother she would shape her life through a husband and children. Karril hadn't gone to college to prepare for a career; motherhood was to be her career. Her only motivation for working was to pass the time until she became pregnant. She'd put her life on hold waiting for her babies. Can you imagine the devastation she felt at not having any? Nothing in her upbringing had prepared her for this. Her parents never told her there'd be disappointments. She'd been put on a pedestal and insulated, a baby boom princess born into an emerging middle class.

So, when infertility clung to her like a raw, black fog, she had no clues how to wipe it off. The longer she remained childless, the less self-esteem she had. Until now, when she had none, when she was an unhappy woman with a hollow life. No cushion. No center.

I sat at work and wondered how psychiatrists diagnosed a split personality. What convinced them that a patient wasn't just an ordinary flake, but two wrapped together, and then not too tightly? For all intents and purposes I was a solid, dependable, functional staff writer for the *Washington Post*. I went out, reported my stories, came back and wrote them. I never missed a deadline. Whatever the pieces needed—facts, order, context, compassion, understanding, humor—I patched in. I could change gears on the fly, go from an accordion convention to a punk Congressman to an old song and dance man like Pinky Lee whom I'd interviewed yesterday, without breaking stride. I tried to be witty and charming in the office. For the past week I had been acutely sensitive to how I was being perceived by my co-workers, and to the best of my knowledge I hadn't gotten any odd stares. Apparently nobody thought I was acting strangely. Yet here I was juggling this act in one hand and a black market baby sale in the other, and my insides felt like scrambled eggs. I guess you can fool all the people some of the time. Maybe I'd blown the career. Maybe I should have chucked reporting and joined the CIA.

My musings were interrupted by a phone call from Les Scherr, the lawyer whom Sidney Sachs had recommended. I outlined the adoption in the vaguest terms, making sure to avoid even a hint of money or scandal, and set up an appointment with him for the next morning.

The instant that I hung up with Scherr, before I even had enough time to feel crummy about having deceived him, the phone rang again. It was Deborah Luxenberg. She was reversing her field, telling me that despite the $15,000 payment, she might be able to take the case. "I spoke with an attorney who has handled some of these things," she said. "He tells me that the court will follow the laws where the child is born. Even if the relative who arranged the adoption isn't a member of the immediate family, and even if there is a transfer of money, it's possible that if New York doesn't have a similar Baby Brokers law that the adoption could go through. I'm told that the D.C. court will not look into the place-

Wednesday, July 15

ment procedure. It will follow New York law."

Luxenberg was a lawyer, and she was getting paid to know these things. Adoption law did differ, state by state. Arthur had said essentially the same thing, that it was possible that this kind of adoption might be legal in some jurisdictions. But I found it difficult to believe that it was permissible to pay $15,000 for a baby anywhere in this country. It sounded so bizarre that I decided to withhold this tidbit from Karril and not raise her hopes prematurely. And I certainly had no intention of saying word one about the money to Scherr. Still, I admit I was feeling pretty good about what I'd heard, feeling like maybe God was good, and we had a legitimate shot at this thing.

And then I got a call which pleased me even more than the others. Because it spoke to the dark side of me. It was from my friend, Ted Beitchman, and it was about Grace Zimmer and the possibility of the proverbial smoking gun.

"Your hunch was right," Ted said. "My relatives in Clifton know the Zimmers very well. It turns out that my cousin is about the same age as Grace. Grace works as a secretary in a medical building, and her husband is an exterminator."

"Exterminator? Talk about your class acts. 'Hi, Zimmer's the name; bugs are my game. If it crawls, swarms, or flies, I'll make sure it dies.' You go to school for that, or just hang around your local garbage dump for a couple of summers? I mean, nice work if you can get it, huh?"

"Calm down. My aunt says they're very nice folks and very good parents."

"Great. Maybe we should nominate them for the Nobel Prize in roach control."

"Now here's something you might like. I had to tell

129

Wednesday, July 15

my aunt why I was calling about these people, and I told her about the money. I asked if the Zimmers seemed to live above their means. She didn't think they could be making too much money, her being a secretary and him not owning the company. She said they had a nice house, but nothing special. But when she thought about it she said, 'Grace does wear very expensive jewelry. I'd love to buy jewelry like hers, but I don't have that kind of money.'"

I sat silently, just letting the inference shower me like pennies from heaven.

"You like that, don't you?" Ted asked.

"Like it? I love it. I love thinking that I'm giving this bitch a down payment on the Hope Diamond." I paused for effect. "Then again, I wonder if the IRS might be interested in how the little lady got her rocks."

Thursday, July 16

I was twenty and Karril was eighteen when we met. My college roommate's parents owned a summer camp in the Pocono Mountains in northeastern Pennsylvania—Tioga, an Indian word presumably meaning "child of rich parents"—and they hired me to be a counselor.

I supervised twenty-four waiters, fifteen- and sixteen-year-old boys, the senior group of paying campers, and ran the dining room operations, making sure the meals were delivered and removed efficiently and the spills were wiped up promptly. Which is to say I was a low-rent maitre d'. I didn't prepare the food, but because I watched it done, I rarely ate it. I knew that my waiters, as generations of camper-waiters had done before them, put laxative in the chocolate pudding, drool in the iced tea, and boogers in the chow mein. I admit that I condoned such behavior in the spirit of historical linkage. Because camp life is different from real life. It has its own natural law, its own rhythm, its own gravity. Those of you who have been to camp know it as a safe harbor from the choppy sea of adolescence. The shaving cream fights, the beer cans cooling in the toilet tanks, the midnight raids, the ad hoc usage of live frogs as roller-hockey pucks, that's all part of camp life. That's tradition. You wouldn't want to mess around with tradition even if your roommate's parents owned the place. Let's be real;

you can always get another roommate. But once your youth is gone, it's gone forever.

    The dining room area at Camp Tioga was divided into boys' side and girls' side. And the first day of camp I was on girls' side, going from table to table trying to make sure that the right number of campers and counselors were seated at the right tables. I reached one table where there were supposed to be two counselors and ten campers from the Juniors group, twelve year olds. I looked around and saw a bunch of girls and a woman in her mid-forties whom I assumed was a member of the married staff, trading her summer salary so that her children could attend camp at a cut rate.

    "My chart says there's supposed to be two counselors here," I said. "I only see one. Where's the other?"

    One of the campers said, "She's over there," pointing to the far end of the table, right side, closest to the window.

    I looked over at a slender girl in a sundress, with large, fawn-brown eyes and thick brown hair, parted into pigtails and wrapped by orange ribbons. A very cute girl, I thought, but far too young to be a counselor. A kid.

    I pointed at her.

    "You're a counselor?" I asked in disbelief.

    She nodded. Her face was beginning to flush in embarrassment.

    Displaying my usual tact and savoir faire, I said, "You've got to be kidding me. You look twelve years old."

    Her cheeks were the color of paprika.

    "I'm eighteen," she said.

    I can't say that it was love at first sight, but it certainly was deep-like, at least on my side. It took me nearly two weeks to reverse the first impression I'd made and get her to agree to go out with me. I'd never had a camp

Thursday, July 16

romance last through Labor Day before. When we were still going strong by Thanksgiving I knew this one was special. Each person you love has something distinctive, something extraordinary, something so memorable you can't get it out of your mind. A look. A touch. A mannerism. A scent. A laugh. Karril's gift was her smile. Wide as an ocean and deep as a river, come rain or come shine. Every time I saw it, I melted.

I was twenty-three and Karril was twenty-one when we married. Down the road would be children. At least two, possibly three. But there was no rush. We had our whole lives ahead of us.

I was twenty-five and Karril was twenty-three when she stopped taking the pill. We assumed that she would become pregnant within the year. Why shouldn't we? When the year passed without Karril conceiving I wasn't particularly concerned. At the time I didn't know that a couple was clinically diagnosed as infertile after one year of trying and failing to conceive. I just figured that some people get there quicker than others; my parents had been married almost eight years before they had me. But after a second year passed without Karril becoming pregnant I suggested that we seek medical help. Karril found a gynecologist who specialized in infertility, and he instructed her to begin taking her temperature on a daily basis and to record the exact degrees on a basal temperature chart. The theory was that the chart would graph her menstrual cycle and reveal the optimal time for the intercourse that would lead to conception. This often succeeds with women who have regular cycles. Unfortunately, Karril had never been regular, and consequently her charts never displayed the standard plot of peaks and valleys that could make a gynecologist confident of pinpointing the period of ovulation.

We tried our best to make love at what we thought

Thursday, July 16

was the propitious time, although the pressure for performance drained much of the love from the act. It was more like a laboratory experiment, and sometimes no more emotionally satisfying than cleaning the oven.

I was twenty-seven and Karril was twenty-five. All around us couples our age were having no difficulties starting their families. We were beginning to feel jinxed. We were advised that infertility was common, that 50 percent of all cases were treated successfully; we should have patience and stick to the program. So we did for another year, and still nothing happened. Karril's Crohn's disease was worsening, but as far as we knew it was an intestinal disorder, unrelated to her reproductive system. So why weren't babies coming?

I was twenty-eight and Karril was twenty-six. The clock was ticking. I don't know precisely when I first mentioned adoption, but I know Karril wanted nothing to do with it. She wanted to be a natural mother; she didn't want anyone else's baby. I agreed not to press it, and she agreed to switch gynecologists. She began seeing a doctor in New York City named Charles Debrovner who had been written up in *Time* magazine as a leading specialist in the treatment of infertility.

The first thing he wanted was me to get my sperm tested for potency. It never occurred to me that I might be the culprit, and the suggestion terrified me. I knew Karril felt incomplete by being unable to bear children, but she said she didn't feel less feminine because of it. The prospect of being sterile affected me in a far more dramatic manner. My whole self-image was threatened. I had never minded being physically weak, but if I shot blanks—that would make me less than a man. I didn't know how I could face people if it turned out that I was the cause of our infertility. Suddenly I understood why Karril was always offering to give me a divorce so I

Thursday, July 16

could go and have my babies. Maybe life was a country-western song after all.

The urologist I went to see instructed me to ejaculate into a pill jar and rush the semen to his office to be analyzed. I wasn't sure I could fill up a thimble, which was embarrassing enough. But how was I supposed to get it in there? Maybe I'd led a sheltered life, but I'd never considered masturbation as a form of target practice. Having to get my sperm checked was intimidating already, but this procedure was totally humbling. The night before the test I loaded up on wheat germ and cottage cheese. Honestly. Because I'd read somewhere that they contained vitamin K, and vitamin K increased the sperm count. Look, you've got to take a test, you might as well cram.

The next morning, bright and early, I went into the bathroom as instructed, conjured up a highlight film of impure thoughts, and, as they say, abused myself. The pill jar was a dead issue. What if I missed? I did it into a Dixie cup, put a piece of tinfoil over the top and drove to the urologist's praying that a cop wouldn't pull me over for running a stop sign, see the cup sitting on the front seat and ask to see just what I was drinking at this hour.

Fortunately I made it over there without incident. I parked the car and went into the doctor's office. Given the sensitivity of having to take a sperm test you'd think that a doctor might be considerate enough to hire seventy-five-year-old grandmothers for his office staff. Not this guy. This guy must have been the valedictorian at Marquis de Sade Medical College. Every one of his employees looked like a finalist in a Dolly Parton look-alike contest. After sitting with my head down, staring at my feet for what seemed like forever, I was summoned to the urologist's inner office. I gave him my Dixie cup

Thursday, July 16

and mumbled my apologies for the size of the sample and for not bringing it in the prescribed container. My future was out of my hands now, and in his. Then I went to leave, assuming he would have my sperm analyzed in a lab and call me with the results in a few days. My back was already turned when I heard him say, "Let's have a look."

My God, he was going to tell me *now*. I wasn't prepared for this at all. My nerves started vibrating so, I felt like a Cuisinart in overdrive.

He removed the tinfoil, and with the imperiousness a gourmet chef might exhibit examining a Big Mac, he glanced inside.

"Looks normal to me," he said.

Like they say, I didn't know whether to spit or wind my watch.

"You mean I'm fertile?"

"Seems so."

"And that's it? You don't have to put it on a slide under a microscope?" I couldn't believe the most solemn judgment on my life was being made so casually.

"I will. But from what I can see here it's perfectly normal."

Nothing that I could hear, not winning the Pulitzer Prize, not being declared sole heir to the Howard Hughes estate, not even being told by the Pope that I was Jesus' long lost brother, absolutely nothing could have sounded better to me than what I'd just heard: I wasn't sterile. I walked outside and cried for joy.

When I reported the verdict to Dr. Debrovner he went to work on Karril. He performed a laparoscopy, a surgical procedure to determine if her fallopian tubes were open. They were. But he found that her left ovary was so encased by scar tissue that she would probably never become pregnant from that side. Still, her right ovary

Thursday, July 16

appeared functional, and he told us that Karril should be able to pass eggs from that side. He said there was no reason to believe that her Crohn's disease precluded her conceiving. Again, we were given a specific program starting with the temperature charts, but now including a dose of Clomid, a fertility drug.

We did as instructed for another year, and it was in this year that I persuaded Karril to attend the adoption workshop in Long Beach, just so we might consider the alternative. But we were so discouraged by what we learned there that we tabled the idea of adopting and continued to try for a natural child. By now, however, our sexual relationship had lost all spontaneity. Virtually the only times we had intercourse were every other day between the twelfth and sixteenth days following the first day of Karril's period, when we hoped she might be ovulating.

I was twenty-nine and Karril was twenty-seven. Such was Karril's obsession with becoming a mother, that for years, whenever her period was slightly overdue, even by a matter of days, she rushed to the lab and took a pregnancy test. I pleaded with her to stop torturing herself like this, that the anxiety it provoked was destructive to her and to us. She insisted that not knowing was worse than the disappointment of being told she wasn't pregnant, but when, invariably, the finding was negative, she would fall into a depression that sometimes lasted for weeks. The inability to have children strained our marriage, gorging at the fiber like a swarm of locusts. It isolated us from couples our own age, crippled our sex life, and led us to believing we were sinful. God says, "Be fruitful and multiply." If we couldn't, how could we be in His likeness? We must be terrible people for Him to have made this terrible judgment on us. There were times, I admit, when I felt so lousy about our

Thursday, July 16

predicament that, in my frustration, I hurt Karril badly. I remember closing an argument by shouting, "Why am I even wasting my time talking to you like a normal human being? If you were normal, you'd have a kid by now." I knew it was unforgivable, and I said it anyway.

I was thirty and Karril was twenty-eight when my mother died from cancer. Her death wasn't unexpected, and I'd had two months to prepare for it as best I could. I've always had a semi-mystical notion about death. I believe that though bodies die, souls don't. At the instant of death, the soul is reborn into a new body. It could be human, animal, or plant, but I believe the soul enters a living thing somewhere.

We flew down to Florida for the funeral and stayed there with my father for the Jewish religion's traditional week of mourning. A couple of weeks after we'd gotten home Karril said her period was overdue and she intended to take a pregnancy test. I didn't think she was pregnant. I suspected she was late either because of the stress of my mother's death, or the climate change between Florida and New York. When the test result came out negative, I assumed my suspicions were vindicated. But a week passed and Karril still didn't get her period. Now she was saying she really felt she was pregnant, and she insisted on taking the test again. When the result came back from the second test, it was inconclusive, and she was advised to take yet another test. The lab report on this third test indicated Karril was pregnant.

I didn't know what to believe. Half of me was unconvinced. One test was negative; one test was inconclusive; one test was positive. All on the same woman. All within ten days. But how could I help but think what a divine blessing it would be if my mother's soul had been reborn into the child Karril might be carrying?

If I was confused, Karril wasn't. She was elated. I had

Thursday, July 16

never seen her so happy. Her old smile was suddenly back, and that special glow pregnant women suddenly get, she had it. Whatever horrible burden she had borne was lifted. Dust in the wind. I went out and bought a bottle of champagne for the occasion. Even if I was skeptical it wouldn't hurt to buttress Karril. I felt obligated to tell my father, but I soft-pedaled the news, cautioning that Karril had gone through three tests and this latest finding could easily be mistaken. I was deliberately skeptical because I didn't want to open myself to extra pain in case the whole thing went south. But a few nights later at a party in Manhattan we told some friends that Karril was expecting and their reaction was so thrilling, it turned me around. I dropped my defenses and spent the rest of the evening three feet off the ground.

Unfortunately, the baby, if indeed there really was one, was short-lived. The next day Karril began to stain, an ominous sign. She immediately went to see Dr. Debrovner who concluded she had miscarried. "It was probably a spontaneous abortion," he told her. "Your body probably rejected the egg because it knew it wasn't right."

That was all I needed. I felt Karril would never be able to carry to term because her body was weakening under the Crohn's disease. I viewed this Kohutek of a pregnancy as the ultimate tease. From that point on I was convinced we would never have children together, that we should either adopt, or divorce and take our shots with other partners. On the other hand, Karril was equally convinced that if she became pregnant once, she could again. Dr. Debrovner seemed to agree with her since he wanted us to continue with his program. Another year went by. No conception.

I was thirty-one and Karril was twenty-nine when we moved to Washington, D.C. to start life over, in a new

Thursday, July 16

city, in a new job. The switch surprised my friends and family. They couldn't understand why I was leaving my job as a sportswriter for the *New York Times*. To them, the *Times* was the ultimate; most newspapermen would have sold their blood for my spot in line. I told my bosses I was leaving because I'd never lived anywhere but New York, never written anything but sports, and I thought it was high time to see what else was out there. Which was half true. The second half was that Karril could no longer handle living where we did; there were just too many pregnant neighbors and friends. Women on our block were turning out so many babies, I presumed they got rebates from Procter & Gamble. And in the month prior to our deciding to leave three of our closest friends became pregnant. We simply didn't want to see them anymore. We couldn't share in their joy and, God help us, we had come to resent them. Everything about New York symbolized our barrenness. We upped and ran.

Within two weeks of our moving to Washington, Karril was in the emergency room at Georgetown University Hospital, and her internist was telling me that if she didn't undergo a colostomy soon, she might die. The Crohn's disease was *that* bad. She had a temporary colostomy, and during the operation the surgeon removed the left ovary that was completely wrapped by scar tissue. Eight months later the surgeon performed a resection, and Karril was free of the odious colostomy bag. Her doctors were hopeful she was well enough to conceive, but another year passed without her becoming pregnant.

I was thirty-two and Karril was thirty. Even she was left with little reason for optimism now and in a few months she was making applications to adoption agencies. She was finally dealing with the prospect of not having children of her own. I thought it would be a long

Thursday, July 16

and winding road, but maybe by the end of it I would be willing to accept and love someone else's child as my own. But when Polly Westin told us of the chance to get this baby there was no longer any long, winding anything. Now there was a parachute jump, and we were being shoved out the hatch.

I was thirty-three and Karril was thirty-one when we went to Les Scherr's office to see how we could get him to become our lawyer without telling we were about to pay $15,000 for a baby.

I had all my notes written out.

Names: Westin. Zimmer. Amalfitano. Cavas. Father unknown; mother unknown; social worker unknown. Basics: biological parents said to be healthy and agreed on course of placement; Amalfitano said to have power of attorney. Needs: valid consent up front; guarantee on health of the baby. Fears: What if consent is revoked? Why can't I bring lawyer with me? What about a last-minute double cross? What if the deal is set up to sting us for the money? What's to prevent Grace from calling police and having us arrested for kidnapping? If it's strictly cash, what's our protection? If they ask for the money first, how do we know there's even a baby?

As Karril and I entered the elevator I glanced once more at the notes, then folded them and put them into my pocket.

"Let me do most of the talking," I said softly.

"Okay. But why do we have to lie about the money?"

"Because we do."

My first impression of Les Scherr was that he was a prince. He was sweet, soft-spoken, generous. Before we'd even begun to discuss our particular situation he said he would donate his fee to a private adoption agency; he always does so in his adoption cases.

Thursday, July 16

Throughout his office he had pictures of his adopted children, a son and a daughter, and he volunteered how he knew from personal experience how hard it was to be unable to have children and finally decide to adopt, only to find so many roadblocks stuck in your way when all you want to do is give love to a child who may otherwise not get any.

"I feel very warm towards people who want to adopt," Scherr said. "I always feel that their feelings are the same as mine. They have an inner need to fill up the family and perpetuate the name and the heritage by making a nest with kids. Most people do it by bearing biological children; those of us who can't, substitute by adopting children." There was no question that philosophically he was on our side.

We were still chatting generally when I asked him about a pastel sketch on his wall. It was one of those artist's renderings of a courtroom scene you see so often during television news coverage of a big trial. In the sketch Scherr is standing and gesturing, obviously making an emphatic statement.

"That was the Galison trial," Scherr said, "an adoption case actually."

"*D.C.* v. *Galison*," I said, remembering it from my research. Galison was the lawyer who was convicted of violating the Baby Brokers Act. "You were involved in that?"

"I defended Eddie Galison."

I was intrigued. "Why would you represent someone like that?"

"I wasn't reluctant to defend him. I took that case knowing full well what its implications were, both legally and personally. Galison wasn't sleazy in any way. I believe that he believed there was no violation of the law." Scherr took a long look at the sketch and shook

Thursday, July 16

his head sorrowfully. "You want to know the real tragedy of that whole episode? Galison and the couple who wanted to adopt that baby had all gone to a New York airport together. Galison left them to wait there while he flew down to Washington. He told them he'd be back in a few hours with the baby. Then he got arrested down here and put into jail. That's the real tragedy, those poor people waiting at an airport for their child who never came, and their lawyer couldn't even get word to them. Put yourself in their position and try to imagine what was going through their minds as they waited hour after hour." Scherr sighed.

I knew he'd lost the case, but the fact that he had defended a man who was trying to make more adoptive children available impressed me. It meant that Scherr was the kind of man who'd go the distance on a principle. It made it all the harder to lie to him.

But I would.

I had to.

Without mentioning either the financial arrangement or the terms, Black Market or Gray Market, I explained how we'd been contacted and how we were to go about picking up the baby. I made it sound clean, and he agreed to become our lawyer.

Scherr then told us how an adoption proceeded. First, we'd file a petition stating our intention to adopt the child. Then, the court would appoint the District of Columbia Department of Social Services to conduct a home study on Karril and me. When that study was complete and we were approved as adoptive parents, a judge would sign an interlocutory decree of adoption. In effect, we would be on probation for the six-month duration of that decree. After six months the interlocutory decree would automatically become final, and the child would legally be ours. A birth certificate in the

Thursday, July 16

child's new name, listing Karril and me as parents, would be written. All previous records, including the adoption decree, would be sealed.

"Under what circumstances can the mother regain custody of the child?" I asked.

"If the consent was induced by fraud, undue influence, or coercion. The consent has to be knowing and voluntary. I'd be reluctant to do it if there is any hint of it not being so, and I'd be reluctant to recommend that you go through with it under those conditions."

Nothing new there. I moved on to another easy question. I was going to take this slow and steady. I'd covered too many basketball games not to have learned that when you're the lesser talent, the only chance you have to win is by controlling the tempo.

"Where do these direct adoptions normally take place?" I asked.

"Typically outside the hospital."

"Would you be nervous about getting a child at someone's house?"

"No. I've gone through it that way."

"Would there be any objection to us bringing someone with us when we picked up the baby?"

"There shouldn't be."

I knew I had to get to the money, at least obliquely. I had to give this good man a chance to see what desperate fools he was representing; I owed him his out.

"Hypothetically," I said, stretching out the word as I said it, "hypothetically now, how much can you legally pay for a child without it seeming like you've actually bought a baby? I mean, buying a baby is illegal, isn't it?"

"You can go to jail for it. If it's found out in the discovery process by the court, it can most certainly interfere with the adoption. Then again, I know of cases

Thursday, July 16

where it wasn't discovered, and nothing untoward happened."

Was that a clue for me?

"But for the sake of argument, how much can you legally pay?"

"You can legally pay for the natural mother's hospitalization when she's giving birth. You can pay her doctor bills during the hospitalization. You can even pay for some of her transportation and incidental costs in the last stages of her pregnancy. And you can pay her legal fees. But you can't make any direct payments to the mother, or any payments that would appear to the court as if you paid her for carrying the child to term."

"And how much would that be? Legally, I mean?"

"Probably $3,000. Maybe $3,500 at the outside."

I made sure not to look at Karril. I didn't want to be too obvious.

"So anything more, anything like $10,000 or $15,000, wouldn't be legal?"

"No."

"And anything that involved that kind of money would be somewhat risky, and you wouldn't recommend a couple doing that, would you?"

Scherr spoke to us gently, as a father might speak to his children. He didn't threaten us. But it was clear from the things he said that he was trying to steer us to the path of lesser hurt, even though he knew we'd probably go out and stick our fingers in the fan anyway. First, he said, it wasn't a moral question for him. He knew what it was like to want a child, and he naturally sided with people who did. He knew people who bought babies. Often, it worked out. But he didn't recommend it. "I knew this couple who did it," he said. "I forget what they paid, maybe $7,000. They knew the risks involved, and they said they could handle them. Well, when that

145

Thursday, July 16

child was ten months old its natural mother went to court and claimed she had been coerced into giving up her child. Coercion doesn't have to be money; it can be something as simple as her family telling her they won't let her back in the house if she brings 'that bastard child' with her. The judge found for the natural mother. My friends had to relinquish their baby after ten months of raising him. They were the only parents the child had ever known, and the child screamed and cried upon leaving them. It was a heart-wrenching scene and a rotten settlement. But the judge had no choice. He had to follow the law."

I simply nodded my head. My eyes said, "thanks," but my lips didn't move.

Scherr said he would get in touch with Cavas as soon as he could to get the proper papers drawn up, and he would be back to us immediately after that. He was leaving the ball in our court. But he saw the troubled looks on our faces, and he tried to cheer us. "Remember this," he said. "Even if this one doesn't work out, you've made the right decision about adopting. You've applied where you can. You've taken the first step. I'll do what I can for you. I'll talk to people I know at the agencies. It will work out for you. I know it seems like it won't, but people who truly want to adopt, can. You'll have friends helping you."

On the way back to work Karril asked me what I thought now, and I repeated my standard line, "We've gone this far, let's go the route."

"But what about the money?" she asked. "He said that $3,500 was the legal limit. If we were $2,000 over, okay. But we're almost $12,000 over."

"You got it. And if the mother goes to court to get the baby back, we could be out the baby and the bundle."

Thursday, July 16

For the first time since this whole thing began Karril seemed truly uncertain which way to go. The conversation with Les Scherr had unnerved her. "It's your money, Tony. What do you think we ought to do?"

"Drop back ten and punt."

"Huh?"

"It's a sports cliché. When a football team is in a jam somebody always says they ought to 'drop back ten and punt.' In baseball they say, 'take two and hit to right.'"

Karril's reaction had me off stride. Until now she'd been throwing caution to the wind, and I'd been trying to catch it and put it back in the jar. I took hold of her hand; it felt like twenty years of frozen waffles. "Look, I have no intention of giving them $15,000 in cash," I said. "Either we find a way to do this to our satisfaction, or we get off this bus and wait for the next one."

I didn't expect her to say anything. I knew her answer would come after the baby was born and not a moment before.

I needed to find a pediatrician in Queens with hospital privileges at Flushing, so I called the hospital's pediatric department and asked for the names of some of its affiliated physicians. I got seven names, none of them Benjamin Spock, wrote them down on a piece of paper, closed my eyes, and pointed to one. Dr. Hoffman. I called his office.

"Dr. Hoffman's on vacation," his receptionist said. "But his associate, Dr. Geller, is in. Would you like to speak to him?"

"Sure."

I explained my situation: "We're adopting a baby who is due to be born at Flushing Hospital any day now, and we want our own pediatrician to examine the baby after it's born, and again after it's released. Will you do it?"

Thursday, July 16

He agreed, and I gave him the contact name, Amalfitano, and Grace's number in New Jersey so he could set things up through her. Then I said, "I know it's illegal for us to know the name of the mother, but I'd like to get some idea of what she looks like. Do you think maybe you'd be able to visit her and tell me?" He said he'd try. "And one more thing," I added. "I'm a bit nervous about this, being such a long distance away. I want to make sure the baby you see is the baby we get. If there are any identifying physical characteristics, please let me know."

I told him I'd get back to him as soon as I'd heard about the birth, but I had to go now because there was a call waiting on another line.

Les Scherr. He'd made contact with Cavas.

"He was very cooperative," Scherr said. "The proper papers are being drawn up."

Things were happening too quickly for me to rehearse my phrasing. I had Cavas pencilled in for a piece of the action, so I asked Scherr, "Did he sound, you know, honest?" Jesus, what an idiotic question; as soon as I asked it I wanted to bite my lips off. I must have been nuts, thinking that just because they were both lawyers, Scherr could decode Cavas's ethics.

"Excuse me?"

"Oh, nothing. So, it's going well?"

"It seems to be. He says the baby is due to be born in the beginning of August, so you'll have some time."

"Beginning of August? No. That's not right. The baby is due any time now. Why would he say that?"

"Maybe he doesn't know. Maybe you think he knows more than he really knows."

Was that supposed to be a clue?

"Well, let's say the baby is born tonight," I said. "Or tomorrow. What then? I mean, we're going to have to go up to New Jersey four days after the birth."

Thursday, July 16

"If that happens, you'll get the consent forms when you pick up the baby. I'm going to send you copies of what I sent him, so you can see what they look like. When you pick up the baby, make sure that the forms are parallel. That's very important. It may be the best protection you have."

It was only four-thirty in the afternoon, but I'd put in a long day, and I was tired, and I wanted to go home already. I was heading out the door when someone came over to me and asked if I'd heard the news about the singer-songwriter Harry Chapin.

"What about him?" I asked.

"He's dead. He was in a car accident on Long Island. You knew him pretty well, didn't you?"

"Yeah, I did. A car accident? You're sure he's dead? I mean, maybe he's just hurt?"

"He's dead. It's all over the wires. They're moving the obit. I'm telling you because I thought maybe you'd want to write something."

I did. Over eleven years in the business I'd interviewed a lot of famous and nearly famous people, and with almost all of them, there was nothing between us but a tape recorder. Harry Chapin was the one celebrity who started out as my subject and ended up my friend.

They called Harry a troubador, but he was more of a novelist; he wrote short, poignant novels and set them to music. About taxi drivers who have chance encounters with their first loves and choose not to go home again; about fathers and sons who begin not getting close to each other and wind up not even getting next to each other; about young guitar teachers and bored suburban housewives being swept away in the heat of the moment; about snipers and disc jockeys and true believers, limited men with limited scope. And when Harry died in the car wreck, he left behind the sort of novel he wrote so

Thursday, July 16

well. About a man whose life ended abruptly in its middle. Unfinished. Between the search and the goal, between the promise and the gift. Not yet there, but on his way.

He'd be giving a concert, and he'd sit on his stool, his guitar resting on his right knee, and he'd joke with his audience about the kind of songs he'd written. Harry knew that most critics thought he was a lightweight, and while their judgment offended him, it never discouraged him. He'd blush and tell his audience that when he was a teenager his nickname was "Gapin' Chapin." And he'd call himself "a third-rate rock star," and turn up his energy higher, much higher than his amplifiers, and start singing his songs.

I met Harry while doing a profile on him for the *New York Times* in 1976, a profile in which I said that he sang a course in Morality 101. He loved that. He laughed when he read it, and he had a great and good laugh.

The last time I saw Harry, he gave a concert at Constitution Hall in Washington. It was a typical Chapin concert in that the only reason he stopped singing was because he was told that if he stayed on stage even another minute they were going to have to pay the help overtime; he had already gone on for almost three hours and it was closing in on midnight. Harry did some three hundred dates a year like this. He could easily have been a millionaire, but half of his conerts were benefits, either for some worthy cause or person. He always put his money where his mouth was. I admired him for that.

Later that night Harry and I took a taxi over to the American Café on Capitol Hill and sat around for a few hours solving all the world's problems. And after we finished doing that we drank a few more beers and recalled the afternoon we'd played touch football on his

Thursday, July 16

lawn overlooking Long Island Sound, when I'd insisted I was the better quarterback and he'd insisted he was the better receiver. And he laughed some more, his rich laugh filling the now empty restaurant. Just like on stage, he was the last to leave; they told him if they didn't throw him out they'd have to pay the help overtime.

I remember it was a raw, sleeting winter night, and I remember him telling me that it was about time I stopped diddling around, writing about celebrities, and started writing about people who really controlled the world, the bankers, businessmen, and bureaucrats. I remember me telling him that it was about time he stopped trying to save the world and started selling out so he could become a first-rate rock star.

And I remember exactly what he said to that. He said, "Being a rock star is pointless. It's garbage. It's the most self-indulgent thing I can think of. I've got nothing against selling out. But let me sell out for something that counts. Not so Harry Chapin can be number one with a bullet, but so I can leave here thinking I mattered." And as I sat down to write I wondered where his soul had gone, knowing that wherever it entered, that body was blessed.

Thursday was Karril's late night at work, so I was home a couple of hours before her. I was rummaging through the refrigerator when I saw the bottle of champagne.

"Champagne?" I asked when she got home.

"Yeah," she said excitedly. "I thought we could celebrate the adoption."

"And what if we don't go through with it? Haven't I always told you it was no better than fifty-fifty?" I felt that Karril had abandoned all sense of objectivity, that when I finally made the decision I couldn't count on her to back me up. I saw myself the victim of some monstrous plot, and in my paranoia, I nearly fell apart. "Damn, Karril, you go out and do something like buying a bottle of champagne, and you know what it tells me?" I wasn't screaming. In fact, I was right on the edge of crying. "It tells me you want the baby no matter what. Jesus, it feels like a knife in my back."

"Don't feel that way, Tony. I only bought the champagne because I thought it was a romantic thing to do." She put her arms around me. "Look, we can drink it if we get the baby. Or, we can drink it if we decide not to get the baby. I bought it for us no matter how it turns out. Because I love you."

I wanted to believe her, but I was still scared.

"Okay."

"Come on, it's late," she said. "It's been a long day."

We went upstairs. The eleven o'clock news was on and Karril was in the bathroom taking a shower when the phone rang.

Grace.

"I have good news," she said.

I felt a dizzying surge of heat.

"It's a girl," she said. "A healthy, beautiful girl, nine and a half pounds, twenty-one and a half inches. She was born at ten-thirty this evening. Congratulations."

A girl.

My face flushed. I looked at my hands and they were bright red. My whole body was burning.

A girl.

All I could think was how badly Karril wanted a girl and how happy this would make her; how many times at work she'd daydreamed of the time when she might bring her own daughter to a bridal salon such as this and help her pick out a wedding gown; how that fantasy filled her with joy.

Thursday, July 16

A girl.

I called out, "Karril, it's a girl. A girl, Kar. We had a girl." I hardly recognized my own voice as the words poured out. I was squealing. Literally squealing with delight.

Karril was stunned. Less by the news than the way I delivered it. The squeal. It told her that my inner feelings, the true, gut feelings you can't control, had emerged. It allayed her biggest fear, that I'd resent buying the baby so much that I'd never truly accept it. I knew Karril sensed from my squeal that I already loved the child, and she was confident that I wouldn't despise her even though she was getting everything she wanted and even more—a baby, and a baby girl besides, a baby girl to dress in ruffles and ribbons and brightly colored bows. She said to herself: "He'll be such a good father. He'll be so proud of her. He'll bring her to the office and introduce her to all his friends. He'll show pictures of her. 'Here she is chewing on the dog's tail. Isn't she wonderful?'" In Karril's mind all that had gone so wrong was instantly so right, and instead of a terry-cloth towel, she felt herself wrapped in blissful velvet.

A girl.

"...they put the mother out and didn't show her the baby...probably in a few days, certainly not before Monday...tell Karril not to buy anything just yet...I'm going away for the weekend, so..."

Grace was speaking to me, but I was only picking up bits and pieces of her conversation; I simply couldn't be attentive. I am neither a squealer nor a giggler, yet here I was, totally out of control, doing both. I knew something untoward was happening, and I knew exactly what it was. There was a chink in my wall.

And then, there wasn't. I took a deep breath and felt the heat slacken. I flexed the muscles in my arms. I stood up and tightened my legs, then rotated my shoulders. I was solid again.

"...just gorgeous...your doctor called and it's all set...must be so happy..."

"Hey, that's a big baby, huh? That's great. And healthy too? Fabulous." I was grateful to hear my own voice, not some stranger's, come from my mouth. "Grace, let me ask you something. Karril and I have been talking about when we go to pick it up, and—"

"Her," Grace said playfully.

"Right. Her. Anyway, we were wondering if we could pick her up at the hospital instead of at your house? You know it's usually done that way, and we'd just feel a lot better about it."

"That's not advisable. It's not in the plan." Grace's tone abruptly shifted from bouncy to bureaucratic. We were back to the cat-and-mouse game. I was relieved to be on familiar turf.

"Well, could you at least ask Mrs. Amalfitano about it? It would make us feel so much better. Oh, and we got our lawyer today. Not a minute too soon, huh? And he told me that he and Mr. Cavas are getting the papers drawn up so everything seems to be going smoothly on that end. We're really quite excited, Grace. Thanks so much for this." Then, just for points, I added, "A girl. That's so great. God bless you."

I hung up the phone and braced for the next scene.

Karril, her arms outstretched, came into the room wearing her old smile like a crown, on unsteady, foal legs.

I held her and kissed her lightly on the cheek. I'd just finished overplaying to Grace. Now I was underplaying to Karril. A peck on the cheek is hardly the appropriate response to parenthood after nine years of waiting, and

Thursday, July 16

Karril flinched at the chill. She pulled away and stared at me, her eyes demanding to know why I was acting like this. Where this sudden distance came from.

"I heard you squeal," she said accusingly.

"So?"

"So I heard it. You called out that it was a girl. And you squealed."

"Okay, I squealed. You got me. Now what?"

"Oh, Tony, you were really excited. I heard it. Don't make it seem like it didn't happen, like it was nothing."

"I'm not saying it was nothing. I was excited. I am excited. I just don't want you to get swept away by it." Her smile disappeared. Damn me, I felt like fifteen pounds of guilt stuffed into a ten-pound bag. I was doing what I thought I had to do, and it was hurting her. Damn. "Look, now we know we have a girl, and we know we're happy about it. But we have to be careful not to get too emotionally involved with having the girl and lose sight of the greater issue. We have to keep our wits about us. We have to keep going along with the program." Christ, I sounded like a football coach. "Can't we see if we can find a way of doing this without getting our insides stomped?"

"You *squealed*." She was almost begging.

"I admit it. The point is, we've agreed not to do anything we'll regret later." 32-X, red right, on two. Ready, break. "Karril, don't hang me out to dry on an honest emotion. What do you want from me? Eventually we knew the baby would be here. It wasn't going to change what we'd agreed to."

"But how do you feel?"

"How I feel isn't important. The situation is still the same. We've filled in a blank, that's all."

"Are you at least happy?"

155

"Of course I'm happy. Karril, I said I was happy. I just don't want to lose perspective. It's still $15,000. It's still buying a baby."

"You wanted a boy, didn't you?"

"As long as it's healthy."

"But you wanted a boy."

"So? You wanted a girl."

"I just want to know if you'd be acting differently if it was a boy?"

"Absolutely not. You heard me squeal. Do you think I'd have squealed any louder if it was a boy?"

"Tony, I could be so happy now, and I just don't understand why you won't share it with me."

I watched her turn from me, and in that instant I'd have given everything to start over with her, to get one last chance to make it right, to reach out and hold her tightly in my arms and kiss away all the pain she'd ever felt. Instead I stood brick stiff, convinced that any show of emotion would be a show of weakness. And on the night "our daughter" was born my wife and I slept in the same bed as strangers.

Friday, July 17

In the dream I was lying on the beach with my eyes closed, sunning myself, when I was unexpectedly snatched and tossed into the air. I landed with a thud in a supermarket bin filled with potatoes. I went to climb out but I couldn't; I was completely paralyzed. And when I started to call for help I found I had no voice. Trapped. Totally. Just then a woman in a gray veil that covered her face reached out and yanked me from the bin. Flanking her were two other women in identical gray veils. They passed me among themselves, feeling me, poking me, squeezing me, and when they were apparently satisfied they dumped me in their shopping cart and wheeled me to the checkout aisle. It didn't take a genius to figure out what was going on. I had no arms and no legs. I'd been metamorphosed into a potato. A potato for Chrissakes. I mean, give me a break.

 The next thing I knew, they'd placed me on a counter top in what must have been their house. It was a huge open space, only partially furnished; the rooms hadn't been subdivided yet. By the far wall there was a pregnant sow tied to a toilet. The sow had thick black eyebrows and it wore a sundress and expensive jewelry. I heard it chanting in Spanish, *"Dinero habla, una patata anda"*— Money talks, a potato walks. The women removed the veils, but instead of human heads they had hornet heads.

Friday, July 17

I watched as they danced the bunny hop through the room, and when they got to the hop-hop-hop part, the first woman said, "Fry him," the second woman said, "Mash him," and the third woman said, "Boil him." Are we talking bizarro completo, or what? I was terrified. I tried shouting to them, "I'm not a potato, I'm a human." No good. No voice.

Suddenly the room was pierced by a loud squeal; the sow was giving birth. The women rushed over and held the tiny infant aloft like a trophy, and I saw its face successively change from a piglet's, to the Virgin Mary, to Karril, and finally to Martha Washington. Then the women became frenzied and began howling, "Feed the baby! Feed the baby!" The biggest one seized me and held me tight as the others brought the food processor to the counter top and plugged it in. I saw the serrated blades gleaming up at me and I felt myself being jammed down into the machine sleeve. I heard the blades whirring, and I tingled as they began slicing through me.

We were beyond push now and bearing down on shove.

The child was born; there was a deadline; we had only a few days to make our decision.

Karril and I talked of nothing else, thought of nothing else. Just the baby. The pressure of the decision was making me claustrophobic. I felt myself being zipped into a body bag. I couldn't get any fresh air. I feared I was going to be asphyxiated.

For me, buying the baby seemed so wrong, but for Karril, having the baby seemed so right. How could we do the right thing if we couldn't agree on the wrong thing? Our short term conflicted with our long term. Our moral conflicted with our empirical. If we passed

Friday, July 17

on this one, would we ever have another chance?

This one was here, ours for the ransom.

What a fool believes, a wise man has the power to reason away.

"I'd better call Dr. Geller and Les Scherr," I said.

"Call your father too," Karril said. "He'll want to know."

"Yeah, and call your mother. Oh, you'd better call Polly too."

So clipped, so purposeful, so mannered we were. It was obvious we were hoarding our feelings, fearing that if we spent them it would create an inflationary spiral neither of us could survive.

"First I want to line up a local pediatrician to examine the baby, if we go through with the adoption," Karril said. "Then, I'll call Polly tonight with his name." She waited a moment, then said, "I'm quitting the job today. We both knew it would eventually come to this. I'll work today and tomorrow."

I didn't fight it. "What'll you tell them?"

"That we've got a chance to adopt a baby. That we're not sure it will happen, but I've got to be ready to go up and get her. They know how badly I want to be a mother. They'll understand."

"Just so you don't burn your bridges. You may want the job back if this doesn't work out."

"I don't think so."

"I'm only saying that it never pays to leave a place bloody."

"I won't."

"Don't. Because the odds are that we're not getting this kid. I've been telling you all along that I've got a bad feeling about this whole deal, and you've been telling me all along that you do, too, so what I'm saying…"

"I know what you're saying, Tony. I've heard you say it a thousand times. I'm not quitting my job because of the baby; I know we might not get the baby. I'm quitting because I don't particularly like the job anymore, and there's no future in it. I can't move up. And if we don't have a child, I may as well get started on a career. I told you once before that if this adoption didn't work out I wanted to get another job. I know you're afraid I'm quitting so I can sit home and watch soap operas all day; I don't know how many times I have to tell you that isn't true."

"Okay." I held my hands up. "No fights, okay?"

"Okay."

"See you tonight."

Everything we could do, short of making the decision, was done. In effect, we had declared a truce, so that later we might negotiate a peace.

On my way to work I stopped by the Riggs Bank branch where I'd had the $15,000 cabled from New York. I wanted to make sure I could get the cash in one-thousand-dollar bills. Crisp, new thousands that were markable and traceable.

No such luck.

"The largest denomination we have is the one-hundred-dollar bill," the manager told me. "We haven't had anything larger since the government called in the big bills years ago. You're not going to be able to get anything larger than hundreds unless you get hot at Atlantic City."

How come this never happens to Sam Spade?

In the office I told Harriet Fier about the baby being a girl. Then I called my father. Then, Ted Beitchman. Then, Dan Lauck. Each asked me the same question—

Friday, July 17

"What are you going to do?"

I gave them each the same answer. "I'm not sure."

I called Les Scherr and told him that the child had been born, and that if we went through with it we'd probably be driving up to New Jersey on Tuesday. He reminded me to make sure that the consent forms were parallel. And he once again told me not to worry; if this one didn't pan out, something else would. Had I been a betting man, I'd have bet this was his way of talking me off it.

Fortunately I didn't have to spend all day thinking about the adoption, because I had a story to write. This week had been particularly crowded. John LeBoutillier on Monday; Pinky Lee on Tuesday and Wednesday; Harry Chapin yesterday. And today I was assigned to write a piece on C.J., the orangutan who co-starred in the new movie *Tarzan, the Ape Man*, the Bo Derek bungle in the jungle. I'd set things up beforehand to take C.J. to lunch at Joe and Mo's, a downtown restaurant much favored by politicos. As far as I was concerned, a single photograph of an orangutan sitting down and rubbing elbows with some of Washington's power elite—and shedding on their Brooks Brothers suits—was worth the twenty-five cents it cost to buy the *Post* tomorrow. The text of the piece was simply frosting, and I intended to whip it up light and airy.

Joe and Mo graciously suspended their house rule and didn't insist that C.J. put on a jacket and tie, a rather savvy gesture considering C.J. wasn't wearing pants either. Initially there was a small stir over C.J.'s presence in the place, since it isn't every day an orangutan, let alone such a top banana as this, climbs in to take lunch. Drinks, maybe. But the crowd soon calmed down and allowed C.J. to eat in peace. Washington-

Friday, July 17

ians are not usually nonplussed about fame and profile, living in a city where at least once a day someone in power makes a monkey out of himself.

Although orangutans are generally silent, making noise only when mating or giving their mating call, C.J. spoke volumes with his motions and expressions. For example, when asked what he really thought about his glamorous co-star, Bo Derek, C.J. smiled broadly, as if to say, "There is simply no truth to the rumor that Bo and I are lovers. We're just close personal friends. The truth is that I've got a girlfriend back home in Borneo who makes Bo look like a 4. You should see her swing through the trees. She's the gorilla my dreams."

C.J. was questioned about the R rating that *Tarzan, the Ape Man* received, and he was very explicit in his answer. He took a spoonful of his banana split, as if to say, "I don't see what the fuss is about. I was a naked ape in *Any Which Way You Can* with Clint Eastwood, and that got a PG. You know, when my agent sent me this script I read it carefully, and I am convinced that my nude scenes are essential to my character's development. Believe me, the scenes are quite tastefully done." Speaking of his relationship with Eastwood, C.J. picked a cherry off a mound of ice cream, as if to say, "Clint wears women's panties." Then he scratched his ear, as if to say, "Just kidding. Actually, Clint's a great guy and a helluva doubles partner."

C.J. was asked how it felt to be a sex symbol. He closed his eyes, tilted his head back and grinned suggestively, as if to say, "Chicks dig me. They want to rub their beaks through my long red hair. Sheep dig me too. I get fan mail with little tufts of wool tucked inside. I don't know. I can only suppose it's my pure animal magnetism."

With time growing short, and Washington soon to be sans simian, C.J. said he'd take one more question, and someone asked if he felt he was being taken seriously as an actor. C.J.

Friday, July 17

waited a long time before answering. Then he stuck out his tongue, as if to say, "What I'd really like to do, is direct."

Like I said, light and airy. Any lighter and airier, you could have painted "Goodyear" on its side and flown it to Cleveland.

I had so much fun at lunch and afterwards, doing the piece, that I was able to forget completely that adoption for the afternoon.

But as I was about to go home, I got a call from Dr. Geller.

"I saw the baby," he said. "I examined her, and she appears to be in excellent health."

"Did you see the mother?" I asked anxiously.

"No, but I can tell you that she's nineteen and apparently in good health."

"And what does the baby look like?"

"A big baby, nine and a half pounds and twenty-one and a half inches long. The mother's blood type is O-positive, but the baby's blood is A-positive. Sometimes, babies with different blood types than their mothers develop jaundice, but so far this baby is fine. She's pink; she's on the fair side. Good features. Very round. That's about it. No marks of any kind. Not too much hair. What there is, is dark brown."

"Any genetic problems that you can see?"

"You can't tell that from this type of examination. The Apgar test shows a baby's condition at birth. At one minute old, she scored nine out of ten. Then, at five minutes old, she scored ten out of ten. That's excellent. The delivery was normal and spontaneous; there were no forceps used. I'd say overall she's in excellent shape."

"Well, could you please examine her again? You know, before they release her from the hospital?"

Friday, July 17

"Be glad to."

I knew I had to tell Karril that Geller had seen the baby and given such a glowing report. But I didn't really want to. I didn't want to get into the position where all the news was good. I didn't want to run the risk that Karril would get so fired up about the baby that I wouldn't be able to sell her on the final plan. Not that I had the final plan yet; I still had to come up with it. Before I could do that though, I had to make sure I could accept this baby as my own. If I couldn't, there was no need for a plan.

I was disturbed by my manner on the phone with Dr. Geller. I'd conducted our conversation like a background check for a story; I hadn't hesitated to treat the baby as a subject on whom I was collecting facts. I knew damned well that the night before I had squealed with delight at learning of the birth of a girl, but in reconstructing my wall I'd apparently sealed off my emotions like in Edgar Allan Poe's "Cask of Amontillado." As long as I depersonalized her, referred to her simply as "the baby," I felt nothing. But when I put a face on her, gave her shape and form, when I pictured myself doing exactly what Karril said I'd do—taking her to the office, introducing her to my friends, showing her off—then I wanted her very, very much. If there were no strings attached to this adoption I had no doubt that I would go through with it eagerly.

But there were. And I had to decide if I wanted the baby for a price. And if I did, at what price? Or, would it be at *any* price? I couldn't separate the baby from the money. For me, the money was the critical mass, and its psycho-emotional side effects were the fallout. Was the baby worth it?

Faced with making a subjective judgment I did what

Friday, July 17

any reporter would—I manufactured an objective structure through which to filter the considerations. The List Approach. I took out my yellow legal pad, divided the top page into two columns, labelled one "pro" and the other "con," and set about cataloguing the arguments.

Pro: There was no question but that the sellers were making a profit off our misery. But they hardly held the franchise on grief money. When was the last time anyone was overjoyed having to seek out the services of a funeral parlor or a finance company? The reality was that many legitimate businesses, even some honored ones, owed their solvency to other people's misfortunes.

Pro: Had Karril become pregnant we'd have cheerfully paid maternity, hospital, and postpartum recuperative costs. The total expenditure, combining medical charges with income lost through her inability to remain at work, would surely amount to many thousands of dollars. Was it fair and reasonable to deny any remuneration to the surrogate carrying the child we so desperately sought? Was it fair and reasonable to hold her to a moral standard which condemned the act of having a child out of wedlock as sinful and punished it by allowing no financial recompense?

Pro: We were receiving a child, and the sellers were receiving a fee. Given mutual agreement, and no charge of victimization from either side, and assuming the adopted child went to good and loving parents, where were grounds for objection?

Pro: Had we been accepted by a private adoption agency we would have had to pay fees both for the mandatory home study by a social worker and the placement of the child. We might even have been encouraged to make a charitable contribution to the agency. If the issue was selling, wasn't the private agency in the selling

Friday, July 17

business? Wasn't the distinction between buying a baby from a private source or a licensed private adoption agency merely one of semantics?

Pro: The time would come when my daughter would want to know the circumstances of her adoption. Might she not be pleased to learn that I wanted her so much that I was willing to spend such a mighty sum to get her, that for the life of me I couldn't think of anything nicer to spend the money on?

Con: Selling a baby is absolutely and irrevocably reprehensible. This is a human being we're talking about, not a toaster. To attempt to limit the full scope of this act by characterizing it as simply an extension of the marketplace is cynical and crass beyond comprehension. What this is, in fact, is slavery. A human being has been reduced to a piece of property and sold as such. Where is moral outrage an appropriate response if not here?

Con: The child buyer helps perpetuate a system which acutely threatens a child's civil rights. Granted, in our case the child would be placed in a loving environment. But what about children who are victimized by being sold to psychotics, to abusers, to sexual deviates? The seller's motivation is profit, and its pursuit has historically spawned such horrifying practices as the splitting of twins and the stealing of infants and toddlers. The child buyer thus abdicates his larger moral responsibility.

Con: Buying a child contradicts contemporary notions of altruism and fairness in adoption. The child buyer decreases the overall pool of children available for adoption, and by circumnavigating established waiting lists he, in effect, bumps down all prospective adopters on the theoretical master list.

Con: Even if the immorality of buying and selling a

Friday, July 17

child is arguable, it is clearly illegal to do it. By law whoever is in receipt of illegally sold goods is obligated, upon investigation and discovery, to relinquish them.

Con: How long, if ever, would it take for me to look at my daughter and not see the dollar signs? How could I raise her without constantly being reminded of what I did to obtain her? That I bought her, cash on delivery. That I owned her. Could I ever truly love her as a person, not goods? And what kind of guilt trip is that for a father to carry around? What would I use to rub out the stain? Where can you buy industrial-strength emotional solvent?

I looked at my list.

I read it over and over and over again.

And I came to realize that the issue wasn't simply money. I felt now that I could feel connected to an adopted child. I felt that the joy that my adopted daughter would give me was worth all the money I possessed, and even that was a small price to pay. The issue wasn't compensating the natural mother. If she was bearing my child she deserved to have her medical costs paid for, and she deserved to get reimbursed for whatever income she lost during pregnancy and recuperation.

The issue was profit. I couldn't abide the prospect of paying commission on my daughter. I believed deep in my heart that Polly, Grace, and Amalfitano were each taking a cut for brokering the baby, and I thoroughly despised them for doing so. They were immoral people. And if I did business with them, so was I.

There's an old story, probably apocryphal, about a gentleman who goes into a classy hotel bar, and spotting an attractive, unescorted lady, sits beside her and buys her a drink. Then another. And another. After an hour or so of pleasant conversation she looks deeply into his

167

Friday, July 17

eyes and purrs, "I can show you a really good time for $500." He reaches into his wallet, carefully counts out $50 and offers it to her. She becomes furious. She bolts to her feet, and with great, frosty indignation she asks, "Sir, what kind of woman do you think I am?" The man is unruffled. He responds calmly, "Madam, that has already been clearly established. What we are doing now is negotiating the price."

I didn't want to buy this baby for $15,000.

What kind of man did they think I was?

Karril had spoken to Polly by the time I got home, and their conversation had left Karril more distrustful of her than ever.

Most of the time Polly had droned on about going shopping for baby clothes and other baby paraphernalia. She had again instructed Karril to get a car seat for the drive back from New Jersey. It was a typical Polly performance, replete with promises of bosom buddiness and a lifetime commitment of friendship between our two households.

But Karril was angered to learn that Polly had known for almost two weeks that the baby was a girl, and had deliberately kept the information from us. Apparently the sonogram had revealed the sex of the baby, and Grace and Polly had agreed not to tell us. On one hand the admission infuriated Karril because it revealed a lack of honesty on Polly's part. On the other hand it delighted Karril because it confirmed her suspicions about Polly's true character and justified Karril's dislike for her.

Towards the end of their conversation Karril mentioned that she had contacted a local pediatric group to set up an appointment for the baby to be examined as soon as we brought her home. Karril clicked off the

Friday, July 17

names of the doctors in the group, and when she got to the fourth name Polly interrupted.

"You want to stay away from him," Polly said sternly.

"That's funny," Karril said. "He was the one I made the actual appointment with."

"Don't see him." Polly was clearly agitated. "His wife is a social worker. When she hears about the adoption she might start to ask questions and blow the lid off everything."

Interesting phrase, I thought. *Blow the lid off everything.*

Saturday, July 18

My private sanctuary was the small upstairs bedroom I used as my office. I'd walk in and be comforted by swatches of my past: a huge map of the United States glittering with colored foil stars I'd pasted on cities I'd visited; my college diploma; awards I'd won for my writing; my softball trophies, photographs of me, Karril, family, and friends; framed montages of free-lance magazine pieces I wrote and my by-lined front page stories from *Newsday,* the *New York Times* and the *Washington Post;* a large glass bowl in which I kept matchbooks from restaurants I'd eaten in; souvenirs from travels, like a miniature cable car from San Francisco, seashells from Miami Beach, a toy cannon from West Point, a replica of Philadelphia's Liberty Bell, a peanut-under-glass from Jimmy Carter's hometown of Plains, Georgia.

I'd deliberately organized this room as a cathedral to self, a cycloramic history of me, by me, and for me. I did much of my writing here and when the words dripped slowly or not at all, when I began feeling insecure about my work and needed reassurance about who I was and what I'd accomplished, I leaned back, surveyed the physical evidence of my career, and invariably concluded— I did, therefore I can. It was a process not unlike recharging a battery.

But today I needed more than professional reassur-

Saturday, July 18

ance, I needed spiritual guidance. And I didn't know where to turn but to my mother. She'd been dead for more than three years, but a day didn't go by when I didn't palpably feel her presence or see her face before me. She was my best friend and biggest booster, and without her I'd sensed myself drifting, unfocused and desultory. If only she were alive, together we'd find the way out of this maze. So I sat there and tried to conjure the advice I sought. I gathered the photographs of my mother from the tabletops and bookshelves, set them on my desk and ritualistically arranged and rearranged them in various configurations, hoping that by positioning them correctly I would checkmate my adversaries. After half an hour of this, a sufficient span, I assumed, for the magic to kick in, I stopped. And as time continued to burn, I once again went back to fiddling with my lists.

Option One: Take the baby on their terms.

Option Two: Call them, and try to get them to alter their terms. If they won't, save the gas and tolls. Tell them to shove their terms and their baby.

Option Three: Show up as if everything is copacetic, then surprise them by demanding new terms. Dazzle them with fancy footwork. If it won't wash, turn out the lights, the party's over.

Option Four: If wheeling and dealing fail, try stealing. Live the fantasy. Grab the baby and run.

Each option hung on the same hidden hook—was there any play with the number? Was the $15,000 negotiable? Or was it firm?

Forking over $15,000 was, in my opinion, unthinkable. Not just because it was too much money. Not just because it was unrecoverable if the baby contracted some terminal disease or suffered some latent, crippling, congenital defect. Not just because it compromised the integrity of a legal adoption. But because it was *immoral*.

Saturday, July 18

The psychological possibility that any adopted child might symbolically remind us of our own infertility was depressing enough to contemplate. Why add to it by having a child who would also symbolize postage due? Stealing the baby was pure romance. Like the political button I favored in the late sixties when I played at being a radical, the one that threatened, "By Any Means Necessary." Realistically, both the button and the snatch were insane. I could count on help from Ted Beitchman and Dan Lauck, but I couldn't ask them to be accomplices in kidnapping, which is what it would be. They'd have to go to the transfer site in separate cars, giving me three cars to play with, one for the getaway and the others to decoy. I'd do a Three-Car Monte, shifting the kid from car to car to car, then sending each one off in a different direction. Grace would never know which one to chase. But I'd need *muy buena suerte*. Grace would have to trust me so implicitly that she wouldn't bring any backup to the site. With $15,000 riding, if she had even half a brain she couldn't afford *any* confidence in my goodwill. And if by some miracle we pulled if off, and if by a second miracle she didn't call the police because she was knee-deep in baby selling, and if by a third miracle she didn't try a re-kidnap, we still wouldn't ever be able to adopt the kid legally because we couldn't risk going to court and being discovered as felons. And where could we go and feel truly safe? How does a journalist hide if his livelihood depends on keeping his name in print?

Whenever I thought about grabbing the baby I flashed on the savviest piece of graffiti I'd ever read: it was on a huge sea rock near the lighthouse off Montauk Point, the easternmost tip of Long Island. Nothing but ocean between there and Europe, and someone with a socio-

Saturday, July 18

pathic sense of brotherhood had spray painted the question—"Where you gonna run to now, Whitey?"

Bargaining over the phone was simply stupid and half-assed. It reminded me of the definition of the liberal Republican: someone who sees a man drowning fifteen feet offshore and throws out a life preserver on a ten-foot cord.

No. If there was any chance of negotiating, it had to be attempted on site, face-to-face, just between us and Grace. And Amalfitano if she showed up. I had two alternative financing packages in mind. In the first I'd offer a lump sum of $5,000, which I thought was a reasonable payment given how much it would actually cost us to have our own natural child. Since we sought to approximate having a child as closely as possible, it was only fair to consider the real costs of pregnancy and delivery. And I'd have no reluctance going to court and petitioning for a legal adoption based on $5,000 worth of legitimate costs. If she didn't go for that I'd offer to put $5,000 down and sent the rest after the adoption was declared final; we'd contracted for an adoption, not merely temporary custody. I'd throw their own line back at them—it's based on faith. If they were dumb enough to believe, it was their problem. Backed to the wall I'd go as high as $7,500. From a strategy standpoint, the extra $2,500 might make them think they were getting a good deal. From a moral standpoint, I was still halving their profit margin.

I needed to persuade them we'd be the finest set of parents the baby could have and if they placed the baby with anyone else they'd have to own up to the fact that they cared less for the baby's welfare than for the cash they'd receive. I hoped that judgment would prove unsavory even to them. As a last resort I even considered

Saturday, July 18

trying to bully them into an agreement by threatening to expose their whole slimy scheme in print. Names, dates and places. Admittedly, it's a problem ethically, using my journalistic connections as a weapon—and I didn't do it. But I considered it. In any case, if I left with the baby I wasn't leaving behind more than $7,500. That was my limit. I wasn't George Steinbrenner, and this baby wasn't Dave Winfield. You have to have a bottom line or you're not negotiating, you're just stalling, and eventually they'll recognize you for the patsy you are.

That was my plan.

It had the makings of a made-for-TV movie. As long as I controlled the characters and the dialogue it would work. They'd get religion. We'd get the baby. And the money would be forgotten.

Unfortunately, this wasn't Hollywood. And this was the choice I was giving them: negotiate with us and come away with $7,500. Or, stand pat, keep the baby and sell it for $15,000 to someone else.

So, what were my chances?

Somewhere between slim and none.

It was obvious I had absolutely no control over the sellers, so I turned my attention towards Karril. Like many insecure people I sought to manage others to substitute for my inability to manage myself. As such, much of my behavior was based on countervalence. For example, to neutralize the painc that set in whenever I had to confront an unknown I tried to make myself unavailable for duty by saturating my life with small, detailed tasks, full of sound and fury signifying nothing. That way I not only avoided new situations, but by following a synthetic regimen I wove a cloth of order and competence. No one who saw me function with such precision could ever suspect that it was an illusion,

Saturday, July 18

that at core I saw myself as totally ineffectual.

Making lists, collecting matchbooks only from restaurants I'd eaten in, wearing a certain pair of underwear only on airplane flights, squeezing the grapefruits only after I'd completed my exercise routine, reaching down to touch the top step on the staircase on the way up but never on the way down, these weren't randomly acquired habits but specific ritualistic obsessions, the moveable parts of my coping mechanism. My phobic responses to flying, to meeting new people in social situations, to going out without an itemized itinerary reflected my anxiety at being placed in settings where I not only had no control of events, but where I couldn't even compensate through compulsive planning.

The reality of this adoption was that it was new and chancy and manipulated by strangers, and those factors in combination had pushed me to the verge of emotional paralysis. I had no similar experiences to fall back on, no reference points to comfort and guide me. Buying a baby was a frightening prospect, and I had every right to be frightened by it. All I wanted was out. But I was too insecure to admit my fears to Karril. Instead, I tried to maneuver her into voting my proxy. I was scared, and I wanted to lay it off on her.

I could hardly ask her to take it on trust that we'd be better off passing on this baby. Who died and named me Solomon? And what was the sugar for Karril? It would seem to her like another loyalty oath, and she had already taken too many of those. No, she had to come to the decision herself and be comfortable with it, or it would not work.

I knew she didn't care about the money or the morality as much as I did, but I also knew she was vulnerable to the threat of a protracted seige. That at some future date

Saturday, July 18

the natural mother or the court, screaming foul, might seek to rip the child from us. Karril would not be the one to cut the baby in half.

I make no apologies for what I was about to do, nor do I concede that I was attempting to play Karril like I was attempting to play Polly, Grace, and Amalfitano. I was being Machiavellian with them; they were curs and deserved no better. But I loved my wife, and I never stopped believing that one way or the other we were going to be victimized. So the laws of manipulation didn't apply as harshly. I saw it as my responsibility to persuade Karril to commit an act of short-term psychological violence upon herslf in order to avoid committing an act of long-term psychological violence upon herself.

The first rule of poker is not to throw good money after bad.

It was now a matter of how best to cut our losses.

That afternoon, while Karril was at work finishing up her final day there, I had a long telephone conversation with Ted Beitchman, and two questions came up which made me uncomfortable.

"Do you really want this child?" he asked.

"I want a child, yes," I said. "I want a child very badly. But the way it is now, with the money and the lying, I can't honestly say that I want *this* child, no."

"I know how much Karril wants a child, and I know things haven't been going well lately for you two. Are you getting this child to save your marriage?"

"I'm not. But I know that Karril wants a kid more than I do. She doesn't just feel unfulfilled without one; I think she actually feels *unworthy*. The thing is, she doesn't have the other outlets I do. She's got no hobbies,

Saturday, July 18

no career. She doesn't have anything that makes her feel good about herself, and she's pinned the whole bundle on being a mother. I mean, she tells me not to buy her this kid like I'd buy her a car or pair of diamond earrings, but I don't know if she'll stick around if the deal falls through. If she takes it out on me, if she sees me as the villain, the one who set her up for a fall, she may well split. I'd like to believe that this baby isn't essential to our marriage, but I really don't know."

"Well, you damned well ought to know, and you damned well ought to spend the next few days finding it out. For once in your life, Tony, you should be completely honest with yourself and your wife. Don't you think you owe it to your marriage to sit down and hash this thing out, no matter how long it takes, no matter how much pain is involved?"

"You're not my father, so don't lecture me."

"Someone has to. You don't have the slightest idea what Karril's all about."

"Oh, but you do, huh?"

"I know you don't give her enough credit. She's smarter than you think, and she's stronger than you think. She won't leave if you tell her your true feelings about the baby, she'll only leave if you continue to play her like a Ping-Pong ball."

"She tell you that?"

"No. I've seen that. What she told me was that she loved you, but she thinks you hide your emotions from her. And you know what? She's right."

"Thanks for the session, Dr. Freud. Look, I'm in a negative cash flow right now. Will you take Visa?"

"You can make jokes if you want, but the fact is that if you don't want the baby, and you get it just for Karril, you'll never respect yourself."

Saturday, July 18

Karril and I recognized the need to get out and see different faces and hear different voices, since at home all we did was get into arguments about the adoption. So that night we attended a dinner party at the home of one of the *Post*'s lawyers, Carol Weisman. The guest list numbered ten; us, and four other couples, each containing at least one lawyer.

Ordinarily I'd pass on such a grouping because Karril and I would end up feeling like high school dropouts at a Mensa convention. But one of the male lawyers had worked in the Carter White House and another was a fanatic about the Minnesota Twins and Vikings, and if there were any topics of discussion where I could hold my own, even with Harvards and Yalies, they were sports and politics. If we got lucky we might be able to glom some free legal advice on the adoption. And if the legalese got beyond my comprehension, I could sagely whisper, "Whizzer White couldn't throw deep," and ask for my coat.

We were the next to last to arrive, and eight of us were sitting on the back deck, sippety-bippety, when the last couple showed up cradling their newborn baby. I saw them and nearly gagged. Talk about your bad karma. Here I was, conflicted to the point of implosion by my longing to be a father vs. my ethical convictions, and I get slapped in the puss by such an obvious, blatantly egregious, flagrantly heavy-handed lump of irony. As if it wasn't enough of a tease that mother and child sat in the seat adjoining mine, then, with everyone gathered around, making a coo-coo fuss how this kid was absolutely to die, off the charts beautiful, the mother offered it up for me to hold, like a door prize.

I felt like some maniac had stuck a foot-long, freezing-cold needle into my stomach and was beginning to draw

Saturday, July 18

my blood, drop by agonizing drop. Of course I declined the honor of holding the baby. I never hold babies, not even my relatives. I think it will be too painful for me. It's one thing not to have a child. It's quite another not to have, and hold one.

I mumbled something about how attractive the baby was, then stared straight down at my drink and wondered what a horrible torture this must be for Karril. God, this had to be killing her. But when I looked up at her I saw a smile of contentment I was totally unprepared for. For the first time ever in a situation like this Karril seemed neither discomfitted by being around an infant nor envious of the mother. I may have been projecting too much into a single Mona Lisa smile, but I got the distinct impression Karril was confident that soon she'd have an infant of her own to hold. I must say that impression was more than vaguely disquieting.

For so many years Karril had imagined herself pregnant, large and grand like a galleon, ripe and bursting with the fruit of motherhood. For so many years she had yearned for the day when she could ask the clerk at the supermarket which aisle the Pampers were in. When she could stack the empty boxes in the garbage for the world to see. When none of our neighbors could look at her with sorrow and pity at her childlessness. When she could take her baby, not just her dog, for a walk. I knew how often she had envisioned herself holding her baby, cuddling her baby, feeding her baby — the only baby in history who was never, ever messy. I knew how often she'd fantasized about watching her baby take its first tiny steps. About it going off to kindergarten and coming home with finger paintings and paper cutouts and all the things that kids come home with. And knowing all this, seeing that certain smile made me very, very nervous.

Saturday, July 18

When we got home I told Karril we had to talk, seriously talk. We had to come to some understanding about the adoption. We had to be united. And as usual, I did most of the talking. I told her I wasn't going to lie to her: yes, I wanted a baby, I wanted a baby very much. But not this one. Not this way. There weren't any divine signs; the baby hadn't been born on my birthday. Even if it somehow carried Harry Chapin's transubstantiated soul, that still didn't make it legal or moral to spend $15,000 to buy it. Nor would it make the natural mother any less likely to come after it, or make a judge any more inclined to rule in our favor if he found out about the money. I systematically reminded Karril of what she'd said all along, that she didn't want me to buy her the baby as a gift, that she'd be able to handle it if we didn't get the baby, that she didn't like these circumstances any more than I did, that there'd be no accusations, no recriminations when it was over. I told her I'd hold her to that. Without question this was the most important decision of our lives, and if we didn't stand together we were in serious trouble. "The thing is, we're like Siamese twins here. If we start hacking away at each other, and the cuts go too deep, it won't just be one of us who dies, it'll be both." Finally I asked if our marriage depended on us getting this child.

The first rule of direct examination is never ask a witness, especially a potentially hostile witness, any questions to which you don't already know the answer. Karril looked at me with a chill that could have freeze-dried the lava from Mt. Vesuvius and said, "I don't know. It might."

Sunday, July 19

I'd always seemed golden.

At three, I could read; at five, I knew the capital cities of all forty-eight states; at seven, I was skipped from the first to the second grade; at twelve, I could make ten straight shots from the top of the circle and hit crosscourt backhand winners from behind the baseline; at fourteen, I had grown to be six feet tall, six inches taller than my father; at sixteen, I graduated with honors from high school; at twenty, I graduated with honors from college; at twenty-one, I was hired as a staff reporter on the nation's third-largest afternoon newspaper; at twenty-three, I married a beautiful woman; at twenty-four, I bought a house; at twenty-six, *Time* magazine named me one of the best sportswriters in the country.

It began to tarnish when Karril and I couldn't bear children.

Then, my mother died.

Then, Karril needed the colostomy.

And now this, this outlandish opportunity to buy a baby. I felt no joy, no wondrous anticipation at the prospect. Only anger. Anger at the biological roll of the dice that forced us to grovel at the feet of each and every adoption source. Anger at the agency system that made us a target for sleazoid Black Market profiteers. Anger at a society which valued the accidental act of reproduction but discounted the heartfelt desire to nurture.

For almost two weeks now I'd been coming to appreciate how, once set in motion, events ultimately create their own pace independent of their participants, how spontaneous dynamics overwhelm the most meticulous of plans. I saw it all around us because it was happening to us. We'd been caught in a psychodramatic arcade and been bounced around like pinballs.

Karril and I were in pain, either mental or physical, almost continuously. Her legs ached; her last few days at work she could hardly stand. Her Crohn's disease hadn't flared yet but I was sure it would. My chest thumped. My head throbbed. My whiskers suddenly stopped growing; I'd developed a circular bald patch, about the size of a silver dollar, on the left side of my jaw and neck that was so smooth and pale it seemed to have been stored underground.

My plan was a farce, and I knew it. As strongly as I wanted a child, however honestly I'd squealed at learning of the birth of my daughter, just who did I think I was kidding? I couldn't bluff them. They were showing aces over, and I was holding a jack-high nothing. All my facts and my lists were irrelevant. They may have given me comfort, but they certainly hadn't given me an answer. You can't objectify subjectivity; you're talking apples and oranges. In the end my decision wouldn't tip on plusses and minuses, but on *feel*. Did this adoption feel right? It hadn't twelve days ago when I first heard about it. And it didn't now. The only thing that had changed was time.

Everything was falling apart. Our dream of becoming parents. Our health. Our love. Our marriage. And I was so scared because I couldn't hold any of them together. I'd tried the only way I knew, by force. But the harder I'd leaned into it, the more it cracked. What good would

Sunday, July 19

it do me if all I had left of my hopes were jagged chips? I couldn't do it alone, and I wasn't doing it just with Karril. There were too many disappointments to overcome, too many frustrations, too many lies, too much distrust. The wiring between us was stripped bare. We were one spark away from an electrical fire, and desperate for insulation.

Dan Lauck was our house guest.

In retrospect, I take it as a divine sign.

He wouldn't play favorites. I wouldn't lie to him, or lie in front of him. More importantly, I wouldn't try to intimidate Karril psychologically in front of him. And with me on best behavior, Karril would have no reason to feel threatened and wouldn't go catatonic.

Dan was already actively involved in the adoption so we had no reluctance talking to him about it. In fact, we welcomed his participation. For hours he literally sat between me and Karril on the couch in our living room refereeing. I do not think I am exaggerating in saying that Dan saved our marriage. Without him, Karril and I were history.

He is a dear friend and a warm, caring man, but he is extremely deliberate, and he speaks so slowly that by the time he gets to the end of a sentence you could be halfway through *War and Peace* in the original Russian; if Bob Hope took that long to get to a punch line he'd be in Omaha washing cars. Listening to Dan can be exasperating, but now I was grateful for the time he took because his manner calmed the situation. He went back and forth between Karril and me, a sort of shuttle diplomacy, first getting me to concede that Karril's loyalty to me hadn't wavered during the adoption process, then getting her to concede that my motives weren't as selfish as they appeared, that I only wanted the best for both of us. Gradually the hostility abated, and Karril and I were able to talk directly to each other without trying to score debating points. For the first time since this baby chase began we said that we loved each other, needed each other, trusted each other. We could get through this intact. We would get through this together.

Ironically, it was Karril who made our final decision. Significantly, she drew the line on the money. In no uncertain terms she said that $15,000 cash was out of the question. "Fifteen thousand dollars is clearly illegal," she said, "and paying it on an installment plan doesn't change that." She was adamant. "We shouldn't give them $15,000. We shouldn't give them $10,000. Or $7,500. Or even $5,000. Les Scherr said that the most the court would allow was $3,500, so that's all we should give. And not in cash either, but by check, so we've got a record."

I was stunned.

Not only was Karril stronger than I thought, she was stronger than me; she was More to my Henry VIII.

"I think we should tell Grace that we've decided to pay them only what the law permits," Karril said. "And if she says no, then fine, we won't get the baby. There will be other babies. I really believe that. I just know we can get a baby without having to buy one. We'll work through the agencies; we'll go to Arthur; we'll go to Fern. Somewhere we'll find a doctor or a lawyer who'll know a pregnant girl who doesn't want to keep her baby."

Her whole approach had changed. She was beyond resolute and into *converted*, a witness who'd been washed in the blood of the lamb. I needed to slow her down.

"You want to tell Grace over the phone?" I asked.

Karril nodded her head.

"Look, I agree with most everything you've said. I

Sunday, July 19

do. I think you're making the right decision. But tactically it makes more sense for us to tell them in person. We'll drive up to Jersey and lay it out for them, tell them it's my way or the highway. What do you say?"

"No, Tony, please." She had her hands up. "All I ask you is not to make me go that far; I don't think I could take it if they put the baby in my arms and then I had to give her back." Karril may have learned strong, but she hadn't yet learned stone.

"I hear you. We'll do it by phone."

"Thanks."

I was willing to do it her way, but I had to be sure she understood the consequences. "I just think we'll have a better shot if we do it in person. I don't think this'll work."

She turned her face away. "Maybe it won't."

And in that instant it became clear to me. She'd had the last available seat in the lifeboat, but because there wasn't room for me, too, she was climbing back on deck. She was sacrificing herself rather than cutting the marriage in half.

"Then it's settled?" Dan asked. "And you trust each other enough to go ahead like this? You both can take it no matter which way it turns out?"

"Yes," Karril said.

"Yes," I said.

I reached for her.

"Why, Karril?"

"It's better this way. You're too uncomfortable with the money, and I'm too afraid they'll come back and take my child away from me. Eventually we'll get another baby and it'll feel right for both of us."

"You're sure?"

"I'm sure."

"I love you, Karril."

185

Sunday, July 19

"I love you too, Tony."
I held her so close I could feel her heart beat.

Grace called after the rates went down at eleven. First she told us what we already knew, that our doctor had examined the baby and found her to be in excellent health. Then she told us what we didn't know, that the baby would be released from the hospital tomorrow. Amalfitano would take her home and care for her until we could come up. Maybe Tuesday. Maybe Wednesday. Grace thought it might be best to wait until the lawyers had gotten all the papers signed so we could feel better about the exchange.

"I talked with Mrs. Amalfitano about you picking up the baby outside the hospital," Grace said. "That's fine. She'd like to meet you. We'll all meet at the hospital parking lot."

A few short days ago this news would have delighted me because it played so neatly into my hands. I was right. They trusted us. They were even dumber than I suspected. I could pick up the baby in an open setting without worrying about them stinging us; I could wail away on a Polaroid to my heart's content; I could even set up my Three Car Monte and hightail it off the hospital grounds with a stolen kid.

But now the news just depressed me.

Our die was cast, our Rubicon crossed. I didn't have the strength to get up and take another shot.

Grace said she would call us when she knew that the papers were in order. I simply thanked her and handed the phone over to Karril. Cupping the receiver to prevent Grace from hearing her, Karril whispered to me, "Do you want me to tell her now about the $3,500?"

I mouthed the word "No."

Sunday, July 19

Strange, but after wanting nothing but out I couldn't end it yet. Dreams die hard.

Karril spoke with Grace as if everything on our end was fine. She was every bit as enthusiastic as she'd always been. Bubbly. Girlish. I'd never seen her put on a staged performance before. Maybe she'd learned something, watching all those soap operas.

After a while Karril told Grace what Polly had said to bring to the transfer: clothes, receiving blankets, a car seat. Grace would hear nothing of it. "Under no circumstances are you to buy anything," Grace said. "Everything you'll need will be there. I'll lend you my car seat."

When Karril got off the phone I told her I'd changed my mind about Grace. I now felt that she had been straight with us all along; I wasn't even sure that she was taking a cut of the money.

But now Karril was setting our pace, and she jumped all over me. "Then why was she so insistent about us not bringing anything?" Karril asked. "You know what I think about her offering to lend us her car seat? I think that we'll be driving away with a strange baby, and what if Grace wants to accuse us of kidnapping the baby? All she has to do is call the police, and when they find us, how are we going to explain away Grace's car seat in our car? Maybe you trust her, but I don't. I don't trust any of them."

As the world turns.

Monday, July 20

I worked hard at making this seem like a normal day. I busied myself with the Representative LeBoutillier research. From mid morning through late afternoon I sat at my desk surrounded by clippings, notes, and photostats of campaign finance records, piling them higher and higher, building a fence around myself. But it did me no good. I couldn't find the refuge I sought in my facts because for me, today, there was only one salient fact: sometime soon, although it would doom the one thing we wanted above all others—the chance to become parents—either Karril or I would call a preemptive strike on our own positions and make the adoption go boom.

It was four-thirty when Karril phoned me. She had just finished talking to Polly, whom she'd dutifully called to report last night's conversation with Grace, including the confusion over the car seat. Karril began to painstakingly recreate her dialogue with Polly from the beginning. She said that Polly couldn't fathom Grace's insistence that we bring nothing with us to the transfer. She quoted Polly as saying: "That's absolutely crazy."

I had no idea why Karril was telling me this. Under the circumstances it seemed so incredibly trivial. I interrupted her play-by-play and asked impatiently, "This is your definition of big news? This junk?"

Monday, July 20

"No. I've got much bigger news than this. About other babies out there. I was just getting to it."

Other babies out there.

The words hung in the air like golden thread.

"*Other babies* out there? Jesus, Karril, you buried the lede. What other babies out there?"

"Polly said that just today she heard of two babies who were born in Maryland, one boy and one girl. She said, 'This is really odd. You can go for months without hearing of a single available baby, and now we have three in a week. It's such a strange coincidence. But that's the way it happens. You get these phone calls from people who just want to help young couples adopt.' Polly said she felt so bad for us because we were having to pay so much for our baby when all these Maryland mothers wanted was hospital and legal fees. I got the impression she wished we could have one of them because she said, 'I'm well aware that you've been concerned about the payment, and whether it's legal. I know this is legal in *Maryland*.' You know, Tony, I think the illegality of what we're doing has really gotten to her, because she told me today that she worked for the state of Maryland and she didn't want to be involved with anything that wasn't legal."

"What else did she say?" I was intrigued.

"Well, she repeated what she'd said before, that we shouldn't look at this New Jersey deal as our last hope, that there are other babies out there. And now that our names are known they can put us on the list and they'll know where to reach us."

"Do you think we've got a shot at either of these?" I was more than intrigued now; I was foaming.

"I don't know. Polly said she'd already made phone calls to couples who want to adopt. Do you want me to get some more information?"

"Absolutely. Yes." Call her back. Find out as much as you can. Tell her we'd really be interested in this because we'd feel so much better knowing that the whole deal was legal this time. Butter her up. But try not to sound too anxious. And don't say anything about what we plan to tell Grace. Can you handle it?"

"Sure."

"Good. Then call me right back. I won't do a thing until I hear from you."

Every second seemed like a minute. Every minute seemed like an hour. The waiting settled in my elbow joints and the base of my spine, which suddenly went cold, a symptom of adrenaline buildup. I didn't dare leave my desk; in order to relieve my tension I kept standing up and sitting back down. I looked like a human yo-yo.

At four fifty-five my phone rang.

Karril.

"The boy weighs seven pounds, eight ounces; the girl weighs seven, two," she said. "One was born yesterday, the other today. Polly didn't know which. They're both white and healthy. That's all she could find out."

"Well, do we have a shot?"

"I asked if we could be considered. She said she had already called some couples on her list, and she told me again that the New Jersey thing isn't our last hope."

"Enough of that crap. Just tell me if we have a shot at either of these kids." I was positively rabid.

"She said she'd talk to her contact, the woman who called about the births. But she said, 'Before I can go any further you have to make a decision on the one in New Jersey. I can't do a thing until you do that, and even then I can't promise anything.'"

"Okay, Karril, what do we do now?"

"I don't know. What do you think we should do?"

Monday, July 20

It was my turn to decide. I contemplated our alternatives for no more time than it takes to get wet in a thunderstorm. "We go for it. We go for the Maryland adoption. It's a long shot. Hell, it's probably no shot at all. But Grace and Amalfitano aren't going to cave in. They're not going to drop their price, and we're not going to pay it. So we don't have a prayer on that one. I think you ought to call Grace and cancel. Then call Polly and try and at least get us on the waiting list for one of the Maryland babies. In fact, call Polly right now—we don't have any time to waste. Tell her that we've already cancelled out with Grace. After that call Grace."

"I can't call Grace, Tony; I'm not strong enough." Her voice sagged, like it was deflating. "I just don't want to hear the words."

She knew it was over now. Done. Gone. She'd accepted that circumstances beyond her control had forced her into giving up the baby and the bathwater, but there wasn't any way she could bring herself to pull the plug. The punishment was too cruel and unusual to fit the crime of merely dreaming. I understood.

"I'll do it, Karril. What do you want me to say?"

"Tell Grace what we've decided. Tell her we'll give her a check for $3,500 to cover all the hospital fees, and we'll give them the rest in cash after the adoption is finalized. Ask them to trust us."

I was confused. "I thought we were just going to offer them the $3,500?"

"I've thought about it. You were right. We'll have a better chance to get the baby this way, on the installment plan."

I was grateful for her vote of confidence, however belated. "Thanks. I'll do the best I can. But Karril, I've got to know that you can handle not getting this baby.

I mean, it looks like it's going down the drain, and you've got to be sure you're making the right call."

"I'm sure. I've been preparing for this since we got in touch with Polly for the first time two weeks ago."

"I'm sure too, Kar. I'm sure we're doing what's best for us. We'll get another chance. Good people always do."

For a moment there was stillness between us as we gathered ourselves for the last rites.

I heard her sigh. Then she said, "I love you, Tony." There was a bittersweet poignancy to the words, as if I were going off to war, and even if I came back whole, things would never be the same. In a sense it was so.

"I love you too."

In a second she would be crying. I hung up the phone and bowed my head, waiting for my own tears to fall.

I placed the call at five-ten. My palms were soaked as I held the phone; sweat seemed to be emptying out of all my pores simultaneously. I felt like I'd gone through a car wash in a convertible with the top down.

First I told Grace about the Maryland babies. Next I told her that Karril and I had always been troubled by the illegality of the $15,000. But before I could make my pitch on the efficacy of a deferred payment Grace cut me off. "It is not illegal. I wouldn't do anything illegal," she said. Her voice was cut glass.

I reacted to her tone with one of my own, as flat as a Kansas highway: we were prepared to give her a check for $3,500. No cash up front. We'd give her the balance after the adoption was final. Deal?

It was like I'd slapped her in the face. She was appalled at my temerity, and she snarled at me. "There'll be absolutely no change in the fee. I told you that when we first spoke. The fee wasn't negotiable. We paid $8,000

Monday, July 20

for our son eight years ago. Considering inflation, $15,000 is almost a bargain. They're paying as much as $50,000 for healthy white infants now."

"Well, we're not going to pay it. You say it's legal, but our lawyer says it isn't. And in any case, it's immoral."

"Tony, you decide morality for yourself; I can't decide it for you. It was moral for me, and it's been moral for thousands of other couples. This is just the way it's done." Her voice softened as she spoke. Now it was almost tender. "I'm sorry you waited this long to tell us. We all thought this was a marriage made in heaven."

I wanted to say something. Something enigmatic. Something witty. Perhaps even something profound.

I waited too long.

"There are couples here waiting for this baby, just in case she became available," Grace said.

The son of a bitch actually had backups. She'd played us for chumps the whole way.

"Now I must get on the phone," she said. And she was gone. The dénouement, the last conversation I ever had with Grace Zimmer, had lasted exactly three minutes.

During these twelve days that shook my world, my hopes and fears had been magnified beyond all reason, my carefully constructed wall crushed, my insecurities exposed and my marriage riddled. And now I was left sitting like a mannequin in a window display, holding a phone and listening to the incessant, mournful whine of the dial tone.

So where were the clowns?

There ought to be clowns.

I called Karril to tell her that the New Jersey deal was officially dead, and she told me that while the Maryland deal was still technically alive, it owed its breath to a respirator.

"I told Polly we'd cancelled with Grace," Karril said. "She asked, 'Are you sure?' I said I was. Then she told me again that she couldn't give us a guarantee, but she'd give our name to her contact. Polly said she'd try and get us on the list for the next available baby. It might come next week, it might take six months. She said you can never tell."

"Then these two babies are already spoken for?"

"I guess so."

Maybe it served us right. We'd tried to pull a last-minute switcheroo, based as much on money as on morality. Hadn't we been every bit as commerical and crass as they?

There was no sense banging my head against the wall, thinking about what we might have done if we'd had more time to plan. I let it go.

"How do you feel?" I asked.

"How am I supposed to feel? I feel frustrated. Used. Tired. Angry. I'm stuck here in the house staring at the dog, and I feel like we're back to square one."

"Sure, but other than that, Mrs. Lincoln, how did you like the play?"

"What?"

"Nothing. It's just an expression."

"Well, how do you feel, Tony?"

"I don't know whether to kill myself or go bowling."

"Another expression?"

"Yeah. Actually, I feel like getting drunk. Care to join me?"

"Sure."

"Okay, give me an hour or so for my wrists to heal, and I'll come home, pick you up, and we'll go get invisible."

Monday, July 20

I called my Dad in Florida. I suspected he was relieved that we hadn't gone through with it. He said, "I guess it just wasn't meant to be. But don't worry, when it's right, it will happen for you." I know that's a cliché, but it sounded just fine on my end.

I went through the office telling the people who might want to know: Dan; Harriet; Shelby Coffey; Jane Amsterdam. I called Ted. I called Arthur. They'd all been supportive and I wanted them to hear the final score as soon as possible.

The conversations were all the same. I told each one that I was fine, that Karril was fine, that it had been a joint decision, that we could live with it. I painted as hopeful a picture as I dared. And why not? The losing locker room is supposed to be subdued and reflective, not dead and dying. "Well, Howard, it was a very physical contest, and we came up a little short. I'd like to congratulate the winners on a fine game. Naturally we're disappointed, but we'll just have to go back out on the practice field and work harder for the next time." Better I should say I was emotionally shattered, that I felt empty and worthless down to the marrow in my bones, that I considered this the worst, stinking, most Godawful shafting of my life? I thought not. Family and friends may be willing to absorb your pain, but they don't want you bleeding all over their clean clothes.

I called Les Scherr. I told him the true story this time and apologized for deliberately misleading him until now. Upon hearing the details he said he was glad we chose not to pay the money. "I think you did the proper thing. You could not have lived with yourselves as long as you thought you had bought a baby. I'll do what I can for you. I think you'll make fine parents, and I know you're sincere about adopting. I'll make calls to the agencies

Monday, July 20

for you. It's possible my name will carry a little weight."

That night Karril and I went out to a fancy restaurant, and true to my word, I got drunk. But not drunk enough. Unfortunately, in the morning I remembered everything.

Tuesday, July 28

In the week that followed Karril and I rarely spoke of the adoption.

I suppose we tried to pretend it hadn't happened.

Why run the risk of ripping the scab off the wound? To what end? We were already depressed enough without adding to it.

I was languid at work, withdrawn at home. Karril was thoroughly beat. She'd quit her job for nothing; there was no baby to care for, nothing to fill up her day. But neither of us pointed a finger at the other in anger. Neither cast a single stone. Thank God for that.

I can't honestly say our lives were dramatically different now than before the whole episode began. I'm sure things had changed and lessons had been learned. But whatever those changes and lessons were, their specifics escaped me. Certainly Karril had shown herself to be stronger than I'd suspected. But that didn't mean she'd enroll in law school next week. Certainly I was more vulnerable than I'd let on. But if the adoption hadn't revealed it, something else would have.

And what of the greater truths that are said to grow from shared trauma? Many couples claim a bonding tighter than leather stitches and a wisdom to rival the prophets. Did Karril and I love each other more now? Yes. But did that ensure we'd nevermore love each other

Tuesday, July 28

less? No. Love isn't set in granite, it's a shoreline subject to the caprice of the tide. Were Karril and I wiser for this experience? Of course. But more to the point, would we do it all over again anyway? I think yes. We were still childless, still using but one garbage can, still without reason to ask the supermarket clerk in which aisle the Pampers were stocked. And the longer we remained in that sorry condition, the more desperate we'd become. The next time a child was offered to us, if there was a next time, we might eagerly spend $20,000 or $25,000, or however many thousands it took to buy it. The next time we'd bag ethics and concentrate on reality. And so the only thing I can say for sure about what Karril and I got from all that had happened, is that we got a few weeks older.

I've always felt there are many great morals but few lasting lessons. That along the way we gain insights which seem so timeless that we file them away in special boxes for safekeeping, to draw on and spend like chits when circumstances make them relevant. But our "then" can't keep pace with our "now." We accumulate box after box, stacking them one atop another, until eventually we not only forget which box has which chit, but what made each so important in the first place. After a while it doesn't matter what great treasures are stored inside all this baggage. All we know, is that they're too heavy to lift.

I was still angry.

Not at Amalfitano. I'd never spoken to her. I felt nothing towards her.

Not at Grace either. She'd just done her job as she saw it. I couldn't fault her. I rather admired her ruthless efficiency.

At Polly. She was the one who'd started the misad-

Tuesday, July 28

venture. She was the one who'd gotten our hopes up. She'd had the nerve to come to our home, to inspect us as if we were applying for a bank loan, to pass judgment on us, to insinuate herself into our lives, riding in on the back of a baby we'd never even seen, declaring her patronage and demanding perpetual fealty.

How *dare* she?

Just who the hell did she think she was?

I'd waited eight days, just letting it simmer, and then, this afternoon, after spending four hours with the head of adoption intake at the District of Columbia's Department of Social Services, I called Polly. I wanted her to know we were still out there, still waiting for word on her babies. No matter how badly she might have wanted us to disappear, we hadn't. We wouldn't. It wasn't about winning any more, it was about justice.

"Polly? How are you? This is Tony Kornheiser." I paused to let my name sink in. "Just calling to tell you that we're still here." If only I could will my words to form a noose around her neck. "I was wondering about the babies, Polly. You never got back to us."

"I didn't forget you," she said breezily.

"I shouldn't think you could. What about the babies, Polly?" I kept repeating her name as I spoke to her. I wanted to make this very personal.

"I told you they'd call you if they had a child for you. I don't understand what you're worried about."

"I didn't say I was worried, Polly." I hoped I was making her nervous. I wanted to feel her squirm.

"I told you I was just a contact." She was beginning to sound defensive. "I passed your names along. From now on they'll call you directly."

"Who are they, Polly? What are their names?"

"I can't give their names out. I'm sorry."

"But why didn't you call us, Polly?" I imagined my

Tuesday, July 28

hands around her throat, pressing.

"I can't call you daily. I get news of a baby, I pass it on. This isn't the kind of network you think it is. When we hear of something, we pass it on. We don't call each other every day. I never know when I'm going to get a call. I don't have a baby business running out of my house, you know."

"I never said you did." It just seemed that way.

"I tried to tell you this isn't a formal thing. And I told Karril not to put all her eggs in one basket."

"But you wanted us to trust you, Polly. We trusted you. We thought you would call us back. You said that you would."

"I passed your names along. That's the best I can do. Last month was really busy. I told Karril how strange it was to get three babies so close together. I may not hear again for a year. It'd be the same with an agency. An agency can go a year without getting a baby. There are simply not that many babies available."

"But your babies are different, Polly. You charge money for your babies."

"I told you what we did wasn't illegal. I'd never be involved in something illegal."

"But asking for money in exchange for babies is illegal. It's selling babies, Polly." God, how I wished my words would choke this woman.

"Gray Market doesn't sell babies. Black Market does. Gray Market isn't illegal. Maybe it's not exactly legal, but it isn't illegal. We're not bartering. What we're doing goes on every day. You know, there are a lot of things the courts overlook if the baby is put in a good home."

"It seemed to us that our not taking the New Jersey baby was being held against us. Why else wouldn't you have called back? You were the one who said we'd have

Tuesday, July 28

to pass on the New Jersey baby in order for you to do anything for us in Maryland."

"It will never be held against you that you gave the baby up."

"Well, I just thought I'd call you and remind you we were still here, still waiting." I couldn't resist tightening my grip another notch. "I thought maybe you'd like to get together with us, you know, maybe for a visit. I'd like to meet you finally, Polly. I really would. Don't you think it'd be *fun?*"

"I have so much going on every day working with foster-care review. I just don't have the time. I told you I've passed your names along. You'll be hearing from them when they have something to tell you."

"I don't want you to forget us, Polly. And I didn't want you to think we'd forgotten you."

"I won't forget you."

"I know."

I put down the phone sure that I'd never speak to Polly Westin again.

She was history.

There was a box waiting with her name on it.

Friday, April 23

Over nearly twelve years working on newspapers I've lost count of the number of editors who have sent me out on an assignment with these farewell words: "This one could be a really big story if you get him to spill his guts." The implication is that a skilled interviewer can work miracles; he can coax, cajole, wheedle, wring, finesse, and flush great truths out of the most guarded subject. It is an article of faith among editors that a truly gifted interviewer could have gotten Helen Keller to sound like Katharine Hepburn.

It's a nice theory.

It makes for a nice pep talk.

It's also nonsense. A carefully cultivated source might lead you to fertile ground, provided you cover his tracks. But a celebrated public figure—an entertainer, a professional athlete, a politician—won't say anything for the record that hasn't been well planned. Famous people face reporters every day. They play them like violins. Now, some are "good copy" and some are "bad copy," and a good interviewer can make the most out of both. But the business of spilling one's guts has more to do with timing than skill; you should always know the right questions to ask, but the critical factor is being in the right place at the right time so you can ask them.

In 1975, while I was working as the rock music critic

Friday, April 23

at *Newsday*, I got an interview with Sonny Bono. Sonny had recently separated from his wife, Cher, and this was a big deal at the time because the Sonny & Cher television show was rated in the top ten, and their records were selling in the millions. I knew I'd only have about an hour with Sonny, so after making enough small talk to convince him I didn't intend to do a hatchet job, I asked him the one question that was on everybody's lips—why'd you and Cher break up? Hardly a penetrating question. He had to have anticipated it. I expected him to give me an innocuous answer, something to the effect that after giving it much serious thought they'd decided it was in their mutual best interests to part, but they remained the best of friends. Okay, kid? Next question.

But Sonny said nothing of the sort. In fact, what he said was, "I thought we had a guaranteed relationship. I thought it was a lock for life. We were married ten years, and it broke up because Cher wanted it to. I didn't know it was time for the marriage to end. I suppose it was in her head for a while and I simply didn't know about it. She just said, 'It's time.' It really crushed me for quite a while. I was rejected. I was still very much in love with Cher. She loved me, yes. But no, she wasn't in love with me anymore. I went through all the things that every normal husband probably goes through. You go through the not believing it, the hoping that it's just a period, just a transient thing that'll reshape itself. I think the one who's rejected always clings to it for quite a while, and the other one is out extending from it as far as possible. We tried to keep it from the public because we were aware of our image. The act went on for about a year after we ended our physical relationship. The year the TV show was number one, Sonny and Cher weren't together; she was living somewhere else. You

Friday, April 23

know, a year ago I couldn't have talked about this; I'd have been in too much pain. Oddly enough, I'm not in pain anymore. It goes away. Nature and time take care of it. You do time and it goes away."

Incredible. *The man was actually spilling his guts.* I took notes furiously. When I got back to the office I checked the clips to see if Sonny Bono had ever come remotely close to saying all this stuff before. He hadn't. I was flabbergasted.

Why had he said it to me?

It couldn't have been because he trusted me; Sonny Bono didn't know me from the man in the moon. Was it my newspaper? Of course not. *Newsday* meant nothing to him. Was it my questions? How could it be my questions? I asked him the most obvious question there was. Was it my face? My manner? My approach? Why had he chosen me to unburden himself to?

The answer was that he was ready to unburden himself to someone, and I'd happened to be there. It was the luck of the draw, that's all. If not to me, then to the next reporter who asked him.

I bring all this up because Karril and I had our own guts to spill. We'd been carrying this adoption story with us for so long now, it seemed like a part of our clothing. We'd worn it through the summer, the fall, and the winter. And now that it was spring, and the flowers were blooming and the birds were chirping and the sun was shining, we were ready to take it off and air it out. The next person who asked us—so, how have you been?—was going to get a lot more than he'd bargained for. And that person, as it turned out, was my friend Jeff Lovinger, whom I hadn't seen in quite some time, who was in Washington on business and who happened to call.

Could he come over?

Friday, April 23

Sure. A little lunch and a little conversation? Sounds great. See you in a bit.

Karril and I told him the whole story, top to bottom. We spared no details. The three of us started out on the porch, eating roast beef sandwiches, and ended up outside in the sun, sitting on lawn chairs and drinking beer. We must have talked for four hours. Every so often Jeff would interrupt to ask a question and that would get us going again. And you see, it wasn't that his questions were so good. It was that we were just ready to talk, ready to feel the pain in the retelling. In the hope that we might finally let it go. It was an act of therapy for us, a shedding of skin, a catharsis.

When I got to the part about telling Grace that we would only give her $3,500 down, Jeff asked me if I thought she'd go for it.

"Maybe not over the phone. But I'd always believed that if I could do it in person, face-to-face, I could've finessed it."

Karril looked at me like I was crazy. "You can't be serious," she said. "You didn't have a chance. They'd never have gone for it."

This was the first time she'd said that to me. That meant that even before she made her decision not to give them a lump sum payment of $15,000 she thought that anything less than the full amount would be unacceptable and would cost us the adoption. Yet she did it anyway. I didn't understand.

"Then why did you suggest it?" I asked. "Did you do it for me?"

"No. I came up with that solution because it was the solution I could best live with. I told it to you and you agreed with it, and I was glad."

I still didn't understand. "You thought it was best for *you?*"

"Don't you see? I was worried that what we were doing was illegal, and that someday someone would come and take my baby away from me. This way I didn't have to worry. And in the long run I felt things would be better between us. I was confident we'd done the right thing, and I felt closer to you because of it."

"That took a lot of courage," Jeff offered.

Karril shrugged her shoulders.

"Where did you get the courage from?" he asked her.

"From my gut. From saying, 'Karril, you have to put an end to this. You have to say, "No." Get it over with or you'll make yourself sick. If you say, "Yes," it will never end.' I didn't think I was so courageous. I was selfish. I didn't want the pain anymore. I wanted to get it over with. My life would have been a living hell if I'd gone through with it."

I took her hand. "You know, Karril, I really should have said 'no' from the get. I knew it felt wrong to me, but I tried to tiptoe through it."

"Well, I didn't feel that way at the start. I felt that our prayers had been answered, that it was a phone call from heaven."

"And you never heard from Polly again?" Jeff asked.

"No," I said.

"Ever wonder what you'd have done if you'd run into her?"

I started to laugh. "It's funny, because I actually thought about it. The phrase 'run into her' is right on the money. I'd daydream about seeing her crossing the street and gunning my engine so that I'd not only run into her, but run over her, squashing her like the squirrel she is. With a sympathetic jury I'd get off with reckless driving."

"You're kidding of course?"

I just smiled.

Friday, April 23

"Well, look, you have my condolences. It sounds like a terrible ordeal. But I must say you seem to have gotten through it in one piece."

"I think so," Karril said. "I think we're better and wiser for it. We know more about ourselves. To go through twelve days like that and come out without killing each other says something for us."

I wished it was that simple, that it was twelve days of down and a lifetime of up. It wasn't. We had leagues of sinking to do before we touched bottom. The harder it seemed, the harder it got.

In August Karril went into the hospital for another laparoscopy. She'd been seeing Dr. Richard Falk, a fertility specialist, and he wanted to do the procedure to evaluate the state of Karril's reproductive system. The laparoscopy revealed a mass of adhesions and scar tissue covering her one functioning ovary. She'd need surgery to correct it. Karril agreed to it after Dr. Falk told her it could enhance her odds of becoming pregnant. In the meantime she got a sales job at Saks, but through the entire month of September she suffered severe abdominal cramps. I thought her Crohn's disease was flaring up, but Karril preferred to think it was just a nervous reaction to the upcoming operation.

The surgery was performed on October 1, and Karril's recovery was going nicely. I figured on bringing her home within the week. But on October 4 my grandmother died, and I left for New York and the funeral. When I came back I found Karril in bad shape. She'd been taking Percodan to relieve her pain, and it had so slowed her system that her intestines had become inflamed. She stayed in the hospital until October 12, and although she was fine physically, albeit tired and weak, she was quite depressed. She wasn't ready to return to work, and her mother flew up from Florida to try to

Friday, April 23

cheer her up. But after a week went by Karril was even more depressed. I thought she might be having a nervous breakdown, and I sent her down to Florida with her mother to rest.

After a month, Karril came back and returned to work. But she left shortly thereafter when she was told that in her absence she had been shifted to part-time from full-time, and her position would be terminated after the Christmas season. No big deal; the job obviously had no future. But I got real scared on December 1 when Karril was back in the hospital. She'd gone to see her gastroenterologist, Dr. Lester Marion, complaining of cramps and diarrhea, and he'd diagnosed it as a flare-up of her Crohn's. I trust Les totally; we'd gone to college together. He'd been more than a good doctor to Karril, he'd been a good friend. He never would have put her in the hospital if he wasn't convinced that was where she needed to be.

Karril had collapsed. She had drawn a graph of her recent past and seen nothing but downhill lines. The adoption; the operation; the reaction to the Percodan; the disappointment with the job. Combined, they were too much to carry. She had broken under their weight.

Luckily, my strength held up. Okay, I was angry that everything was dumped on my back. But I seem to have a pretty broad back when someone I love is in trouble. In some ways the load was exhilarating. I've always preferred chaos to calm. I've spent so many years organizing myself to meet the deadlines that it's no big deal to break each day down into specific assignments and take them one at a time. Once I established a routine, it was easy. I think what kept me solid was that I never had enough time to sit and brood.

By January, Karril was back at her old job, selling bridal gowns. By February she had her weight over a

Friday, April 23

hundred pounds for the first time in a decade. By March we were getting to where we could put the whole sorry mess behind us.

"And now?" Jeff asked.

"Now I hope we're fine," I said.

"I think we are," Karril said. "I know I feel fine."

The spring air was warm and soothing. The three of us sat still in the backyard, listening as the birds chirped and the breeze rustled the young leaves in the trees. And then Jeff asked, "How do you feel when you see a baby?"

The right question. At the right time. In the right place.

"Not as badly as I did before," Karril said. "When I see infants at work, I'll go to them now. I wouldn't do it before. I wouldn't touch them. I wouldn't go near them." Her eyes were wide and shining. "I feel we'll get one. I don't know when, but sometime. We're good people, and we did the right thing. God will see this and help us become complete."

"What about the baby you almost adopted? Do you ever think about her?"

I turned away and thought about going to the zoo the other day, seeing the little children tagging alongside their parents, smiling, laughing. I thought of *her* then. I thought how wonderful it would have been to take my daughter to the zoo, to show her the pandas, the giraffes and the gorillas, to buy her ice cream and popcorn and take pictures of her with the animals. When I turned back I saw Karril shivering; it was the question, not the temperature.

"Every now and then I do," she said. "Lately, I've been thinking more and more about her. It seems so many months now. I think, my God, we could have had a baby in this house, instead of being stuck on these waiting lists for who knows how long. It's hard to believe, but the baby would be nine months old now. She might even be walking." Karril wrapped her sweater tightly across her chest like a bandage. "I wonder sometimes where she is. Who the couple is that adopted her. Where they're living." Karril reached into her pocket for a tissue—if the tears came, she'd be ready. "We came so close, you know? So close. I mean, I almost had a daughter. When I think about that I feel very sad and empty. And I don't know when that agency is going to call and say, 'Karril, we have your baby here waiting for you. Congratulations, you're going to be a mother.' I just don't know how long that's going to take."

I closed my eyes and said a silent prayer, that it would be soon.

Jeff wanted to catch the 4:00 P.M. shuttle to New York City, and Karril and I drove him to National Airport. After dropping him off at the Eastern Airlines terminal we headed back home, but instead of going straight there I pulled off 395-North into Lady Bird Johnson Park, a vest-pocket park really, room for six or eight cars at most, on the Virginia side of the Potomac. Looking across the river at Washington you can see the Kennedy Center, the Watergate complex, the Lincoln, Washington, and Jefferson memorials.

"Why are we stopping?" Karril asked.

"Because it's so pretty," I said. "I mean, just look at it, Kar. You know, it's really a beautiful city, even if it hasn't been so beautiful for us. On a clear day like today, it's like looking at a picture postcard." I got out of the car, walked around to her door, opened it wide, bowed, and reached for her hand. "Pardon me Miss, but I do believe my dance card is open. Shall we?"

We walked south on the jogging path beside the Potomac. The daffodils and jonquils growing wild on the river banks were school bus yellow. Azaleas as big as

Friday, April 23

cotton balls and as bright as college students were lavender, pink, ivory, and crimson. Plump magnolias and lacy dogwoods beckoned suggestively in the spring breeze. In the distance I could see the cherry trees that line the Tidal Basin. Their breathless iced pink blossoms, the first signal of the season, had come and gone, and in their place were new green leaves. It seemed everywhere I looked things were busy being born. We reached the Navy Marine Memorial—a sculpture of seven seagulls, joined at the wings, skimming over an ocean wave—and all the strawberry, lemon and orange tulips surrounding the statue, thousands of them, were bold, and clean, and young, and preening. Not yet complacent or overpraised. It reminded me of opening day at the ballpark. A brand new season. No games behind, and 162 to go. Anything can happen.

I was trying to commit it all to memory when I glanced over at Karril and saw that look on her face. You know that look people get when they want to say something, but they don't want to volunteer it? They want you to ask them about it, so it seems like a casual thought, offhanded, like it came on the wind.

"Thinking about something?" I asked her.

"No. Nothing."

"Looked like you were."

"Well, yeah, I was."

"I'm listening."

"I was just wondering about us."

"What about us?"

She stood silent for a second, then asked, "We're going to be all right, aren't we?"

"Yeah, we are. I believe that now."

"And we're going to get a baby, aren't we?"

I smiled. "We're sure going to try."

There was the unmistakable roar of jet engines down

Friday, April 23

river, coming closer. I looked in their direction and saw an Eastern plane climbing strongly, purposefully into the open sky. As it passed over the 14th Street Bridge, the rays of the afternoon sun bounced off its silver tail, and in the reflection I felt sure I saw something like hope, something like a promise.

Evan, if it's a boy.
Elizabeth, if it's a girl.

Tony Kornheiser writes for the *Washington Post*. He and his wife live in Washington, D.C. *The Baby Chase* is his first book.